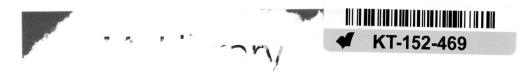

CONTRAST-INDUCED NEPHROPATHY

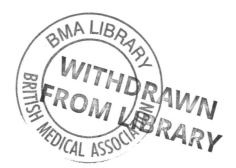

1a	1b	2a	2b	3a
8a		9		3b
8b				4a
7a				4b
7b	6a	6b	5a	5b

1. Left subclavian artery stenosis before (a) and after (b) implantation of a peripheral Carbofilm™-coated stent

2. Severe stenosis of the right internal carotid artery (a) treated with implantation of a nitinol self-expandable stent (b)

3. Aortogram of the abdominal aorta showing a large aneurysm before (a) and after (b) endovascualr repair with implantation of an Excluder™ endograft

4. Eccentric lesion of the right common iliac artery before (a) and after (b) stent implantation

5. Selective right renal artery angiography showing ostial stenosis before (a) and after (b) Carbofilm™-coated stent implantation

6. Right coronary artery angiography in an acute myocardial infarction patient showing a disrupted plaque and superimposed massive thrombosis (a) treated with direct Carbofilm™-coated stent implantation (b)

7. Left coronary artery angiography showing severe stenosis of the proximal left anterior descending coronary artery before (a) and after (b) drug-eluting stent implantation

8. Chronic total occlusion of the right superficial femoral artery before (a) and after (b) implantation of a nitinol self-expandable stent

9. Histological cross section of the collecting tubules and Henle's loops of the renal medulla. These are the kidney microstructures involved in the pathogenetic mechanisms of contrast-induced nephropathy

The angiographic images are from the Catheterization Laboratories of the Centro Cardiologico Monzino, Milan, Italy.

Cover image by Margherita Bartorelli.

CONTRAST-INDUCED NEPHROPATHY

Edited by

Antonio L Bartorelli MD FACC FESC
Director, Interventional Cardiology
Centro Cardiologico Monzino, IRCCS
Institute of Cardiology of the University of Milan
Milan
Italy

Giancarlo Marenzi MD FESC
Director, Coronary Care Unit
Centro Cardiologico Monzino, IRCCS
Institute of Cardiology of the University of Milan
Milan
Italy

Foreword by

Martin B Leon MD

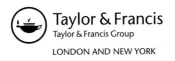

Taylor & Francis
Taylor & Francis Group

LONDON AND NEW YORK

© 2006 Taylor & Francis, an imprint of the Taylor & Francis Group

First published in the United Kingdom in 2006
by Taylor & Francis, 2 Park Square, Milton Park, Abingdon,
Oxon OX14 4RN

Tel: +44 (0) 20 7017 6000
Fax: +44 (0) 20 7017 6699
Website: http://www.tandf.co.uk/medicine
E-mail: info.medicine@tandf.co.uk

Although every effort has been made to ensure that all owners of copyright material have been acknowledged in this publication,
we would be glad to acknowledge in subsequent reprints or editions any omissions brought to our attention.

Although every effort has been made to ensure that drug doses and other information are presented accurately in this publication,
the ultimate responsibility rests with the prescribing physician. Neither the publishers nor the authors can be held responsible for
errors or for any consequences arising from the use of information contained herein. For detailed prescribing information or
instructions on the use of any product or procedure discussed herein, please consult the prescribing information or instructional
material issued by the manufacturer.

A CIP record for this book is available from the British Library.

Library of Congress Cataloging-in-Publication Data

Data available on application

ISBN 1-84184-562-0
ISBN 978-1-84184-562-3

Distributed in North and South America by

Taylor & Francis
2000 NW Corporate Blvd
Boca Raton, FL 33431, USA

Within Continental USA
Tel: 800 272 7737; Fax: 800 374 3401
Outside Continental USA
Tel: 561 994 0555; Fax: 561 361 6018
E-mail: orders@crcpress.com

Distributed in the rest of the world by
Thomson Publishing Services
Cheriton House
North Way
Andover, Hampshire SP10 5BE, UK
Tel.: +44 (0) 1264 332424
E-mail: salesorder.tandf@thomsonpublishingservices.co.uk

Composition by C&M Digitals (P) Ltd., Chennai, India

Printed and bound in the UK by T.J. International, Padstow, Cornwall

Dedication

To the memory of my father, Cesare Bartorelli, who, more with his life than with his words taught me humanity and the art of medicine.

Antonio L Bartorelli

To my wife, Daniela, and to our children, Elena and Valeria

Giancarlo Marenzi

CONTENTS

LIST OF CONTRIBUTORS

Flavio Airoldi MD
Laboratory of Interventional Cardiology
'Vita e Salute' University School of Medicine
Milan
Italy

Antonio L Bartorelli MD FACC FESC
Centro Cardiologico Monzino, IRCCS
Institute of Cardiology of the University of Milan
Milan
Italy

Yochai Birnbaum MD
University of Texas Medical Branch
301 University Boulevard
Galveston,
TX, USA

Carlo Briguori MD PhD
Laboratory of Interventional Cardiology
Clinica Mediterranea
Naples
Italy

Antonio Colombo MD
Laboratory of Interventional Cardiology
'Vita e Salute' University School of Medicine
Milan
Italy

Michael H Duong MD
Section of Cardiology
Dartmouth Medical School / Dartmouth-Hitchcock
    Medical Center
One Medical Center Drive
Lebanon,
NH, USA

Luis Gruberg MD FACC
Division of Invasive Cardiology
Department of Cardiology
Rambam Medical Center
Haifa
Israel

Rajiv Gupta MD
University of Texas Medical Branch
301 University Boulevard
Galveston,
TX, USA

Aaron V Kaplan MD
Section of Cardiology
Dartmouth-Hitchcock Medical
    Center
One Medical Center Drive
Lebanon,
NH, USA

Peter A McCullough MD MPH FACC
    FACP FCCP FAHA
Divisons of Cardiology, Nutrition,
    and Preventive Medicine
William Beaumont Hospital
Royal Oak,
MI, USA

Giancarlo Marenzi MD FESC
Centro Cardiologico Monzino,
    IRCCS
Institute of Cardiology of the
    University of Milan
Milan
Italy

Vandana S Mathur MD FASN
Mathur Consulting
25 Upenuf Road, Suite 100
Woodside,
CA, USA

Roxana Mehran MD
Columbia University Medical Center
Cardiovascular Research Foundation
New York,
NY, USA

Christian Müeller MD
Department of Internal Medicine
University Hospital
Basel
Switzerland

Eugenia Nikolsky MD PhD
Clinical Research and Data Coordinating and
    Analysis Center
Cardiovascular Research Foundation
New York
NY, USA

Pontus B Persson MD PhD
Institute für Vegetative Physiologie
Humboldt Universität, Berlin
Medizinische Fakultät (Charité)
Berlin
Germany

Günther Schneider MD
Department of Diagnostic and
    Interventional Radiology
University Hospital
Homburg/Saar
Germany

Roland M Seidel MD
Department of Diagnostic and
    Interventional Radiology
University Hospital
Homburg/Saar
Germany

Robert Siegel MD
Postdoctoral Residency Fellow
Columbia University Medical Center
New York
NY, USA

Sandeep S Soman MD
Division of Nephrology and
    Hypertension
Henry Ford Health System
Detroit,
MI, USA

Craig A Thompson MD
Section of Cardiology
Dartmouth Medical School/
    Dartmouth-Hitchcock
    Medical Center
Lebanon,
NH, USA

Barry F Uretsky MD FACC
Division of Cardiology
University of Texas Medical
    Branch
Galveston,
TX, USA

FOREWORD

Why should we focus on contrast-induced nephropathy? At an exciting juncture in the evolution of invasive cardiovascular diagnosis and therapy, why dwell on one of our least well understood and poorly treated 'dirty little secrets' of radiology and cardiology? The answer should be obvious to all thoughtful clinical practitioners and scientists as the optimal management and avoidance of contrast-induced nephropathy represents one of the most embarrassing unmet clinical needs in cardiovascular medicine today. Although the syndrome has been recognized for decades, only recently have we begun to systematically study fundamental aspects of pathophysiology, clinical epidemiology, socioeconomic healthcare consequences, and treatment alternatives. As our population ages, as the prevalence of diabetes reaches epidemic proportions, and as we bask in the glory of newly introduced contrast-requiring diagnostic techniques and catheter-based interventional therapies, the syndrome of contrast-induced nephropathy has become the forgotten stepchild, only now beginning to wreak it's ugly head as an important 'dark side' problem which must be targeted and solved in the future.

Importantly, this book, simply entitled *Contrast-Induced Nephropathy*, edited by Bartorelli and Marenzi, addresses another unmet need namely 'exposure and education', by presenting an authoritative text spanning the range from basics, to subtle nuances in this rapidly increasing iatrogenic disease complex. During an era when several million radiographic procedures for diagnostic and therapeutic purposes requiring radiocontrast agents are performed each year worldwide, it remains shocking how few practicing physicians understand the dire prognostic consequences of contrast-induced nephropathy. Similarly, the preparatory management of contrast-induced nephropathy has been a confusing potpourri of ill-defined treatment strategies, with little to suggest that we can truly claim a 'standard-of-care'. This book breaks though these barriers of ignorance and confusion by attempting to separate fact from medical myth with an overwhelming presentation of known data and attention to detail. Respected world experts in nephrology, cardiology, and radiology have joined forces to contribute to this inter-disciplinary compendium. Every chapter is well organized, carefully written and provides clinically useful insights. Moreover, the book is both balanced and truly current, providing the reader with a sense of unbiased data interpretation, reflections on contemporary issues, as well as projections for future management pathways.

Undoubtedly, *Contrast-Induced Nephropathy* is a 'must read' text handbook for all health-related professionals involved in any aspect of the care and treatment of patients who are at risk for this insidious disease entity. Readers will acquire a new-found understanding and respect for the importance of contrast-induced nephropathy, an appreciation of the pathophysiology and prognostic implications, and a working knowledge of present standard-of-care avoidance therapies and management concepts. In short, readers will become better clinical care-givers and patients will benefit. The editors and chapter authors have done a marvelous job in elevating the recognition of contrast-induced nephropathy through this important text and they should be congratulated for this vital contribution to medical science.

Martin B Leon, M.D.
Professor of Medicine, Columbia University Medical Center
Chairman, Cardiovascular Research Foundation
New York City

PREFACE

*The glory of medicine is that it is constantly moving forward,
that there is always more to learn.*

William J Mayo, 1861–1939

Contrast-induced nephropathy, overlooked for many years by health professionals because of an under appreciation of the magnitude and the impact of the problem, has become a widely discussed and debated topic in modern cardiovascular medicine. Currently, contrast-induced nephropathy is recognized as the third leading cause of hospital-acquired acute renal failure, accounting for 10% of all cases and contributing to prolonged hospital stay and increased medical costs. Furthermore, the estimated mortality rate in patients who develop acute deterioration in renal function after intravascular contrast administration may be as high as 35%, and, in survivors, renal function may fail to return to normal in as many as 30%.

It is likely that this clinical problem will assume even greater importance in the years to come. Indeed, an increasing number of patients with some degree of renal impairment, due to the aging process, diabetes, or other underlying diseases, will be referred for cardiac catheterization as well as other procedures that use intravascular contrast agents. Notably, the incidence of diabetes (the primary cause of end-stage renal disease) is increasing by 4% to 5% per year, and the prevalence of end-stage renal disease is expected to rise by 77% over the next decade. Thus, it is not surprising that recent years have witnessed an increasing scientific and clinical interest in contrast-induced nephropathy. Although several publications on epidemiology, pathophysiology, clinical relevance and prevention of this serious public health problem have recently appeared in literature, a text representing a wide spectrum of knowledge upon which to base contemporary preventive regimens and health care strategies was still lacking. This book is the first of its kind to offer a comprehensive overview of this critical topic, with the aim of capturing the essence of the main pertinent issues, and presenting the latest data from a multidisciplinary perspective. The editors have been fortunate enough to benefit from the collective efforts of an outstanding group of transatlantic contributing authors who are world-renowned experts in their field. We owe a tremendous debt of gratitude to these physicians, who found time, despite an extremely busy schedule, to deliver excellent and authoritative chapters at very short notice, and they deserve much of the credit for the quality of this book.

The chapters bridge the disciplines of physiology, internal medicine, clinical and interventional cardiology, nephrology, diagnostic, interventional radiology, and contain an extensive and up-to-date bibliography, which will provide direction for further reading. The book is divided into two main sections of six chapters each. In the first section, three chapters deal with the pathophysiology, epidemiology, clinical features and prognostic implications of contrast-induced nephropathy. Two additional chapters offer comprehensive and contemporary reviews on the cardiovascular risk associated with renal dysfunction, and the effects of renal insufficiency and contrast-induced nephropathy on the prognosis and treatment outcomes in patients with acute coronary syndromes. A final chapter describes the present state of our knowledge concerning renovascular disease in patients with coronary artery disease. The second section is devoted to the most recent advances in prophylactic interventions, including new aspects of the cornerstone approach saline hydration, strategies for lowering the contrast-induced nephropathy risk by selecting a contrast medium based on its physiochemical properties and physiologic effects, and the results obtained from different pharmacological treatments. Furthermore, the role of newer modalities, including renal replacement therapies, innovative systems for targeted renal therapy and possible imaging alternatives to conventional X-ray-based contrast angiography, is highlighted in state-of-the-art reviews.

Books are often considerably out of date, even before they are released. The initial plan for this publishing endeavor was formulated through a collaboration between the editors and Alan Burgess, senior publisher at Taylor & Francis Medical Books, during the 2004 Transcatheter Therapeutic Meeting. A proposed table of contents was drawn up in October 2004, and potential contributors were identified. Letters of invitation were sent to potential contributors in December 2004. First drafts of the manuscripts began arriving at the end of March 2005. During the next four months, a total of 12 chapters were revised and collated, before being submitted to the publisher. Thus, this project was completed in about seven months from the actual moment in which we received the first manuscript, demonstrating that one of the greatest limitations of any multi-authored volume can eventually be overcome. We gratefully acknowledge the efforts of Alan Burgess and his staff, who have created an outstanding text in a very short time. Alan provided us with excellent advice for many aspects of the project, and assigned a superb production editor, Cathy Hambly to assist us. Cathy worked diligently to enhance the accuracy and clarity of this volume. A special thanks goes also to Margherita Bartorelli and Greg Newman for their dedication in designing the book cover and in making it visually attractive. Finally, we wish to express our heartiest gratitude to Professor Adalberto Sessa, who shared his intimate scientific and clinical knowledge of nephrology, and played an invaluable role in improving our understanding of acute renal failure and renal replacement therapies, inspiring us to undertake this task in the first place.

With the collaboration of so many outstanding contributors who are the real producers of this book, we feel confident that it will succeed in drawing the attention of health professionals to the present state of knowledge regarding contrast-induced nephropathy. We sincerely hope that the information herein will improve the care of patients at risk of developing this dreaded syndrome, and stimulate further research in those areas that still need to be investigated. If this happens, we will have achieved our primary objective.

Antonio L. Bartorelli, MD, FESC, FACC
Giancarlo Marenzi, MD, FESC

SECTION I

1. PATHOPHYSIOLOGY OF CONTRAST-INDUCED NEPHROPATHY

Pontus B Persson

Although contrast-induced nephropathy (CIN) is a well-known cause of acute renal failure, the development of CIN remains poorly understood. Several studies have been performed with the aim of shedding some light onto the pathophysiology of CIN. However, these studies have yielded various interpretations with sometimes contradictory conclusions. Although it is but one of several physicochemic properties of contrast media (CM), osmolality has received considerable attention. Osmolality serves to assign CM to different classes. Some of the recently developed iso-osmolar CM are dimers, not monomers as are the widely used, non-ionic, low-osmolar CM. However in spite of being iso-osmolar, they have physicochemic features which differ from other CM, for example in terms of viscosity, which is >5-fold greater than plasma viscosity. This fact may be of considerable pathophysiologic and clinical importance. Several experimental studies provide evidence that iso-osmolar CM produce a greater perturbation in renal function in comparison to non-ionic, low-osmolar CM.

The term CIN indicates an impairment in renal function that occurs within 3 days following the intravascular administration of CM and in the absence of an alternative etiology.[1,2] The occurrence of CIN is usually marked by an increase in serum creatinine by more than 25% or 44 μmol/l (0.5 mg/100 ml) within 48 to 72 hours of contrast administration.[3–6] Typically, the serum creatinine concentration peaks on the second or third day after exposure to CM and usually returns to the base-line value within 2 weeks.[7,8] CIN is generally reversible. Nevertheless, use of CM increases in-hospital morbidity, mortality, and costs, in particular in those rare cases where dialysis is required.

Without question, the greatest risk factor of developing CIN is pre-existing renal impairment combined with either diabetes, dehydration, or both.[9] Remarkably, however, diabetes mellitus *per se* without renal insufficiency is not a risk factor.[10] Additional risk factors include the dosage of CM and type of CM, congestive heart failure, old age, hypertension, route of administration of CM, and the use of other nephrotoxic drugs.[11,12]

In general, any condition associated with decreased effective circulating volume enhances vulnerability towards CIN.[9] Of course, if CIN is suspected in a patient without known risk factors, other causes of acute renal failure, such as atheromatous embolic disease, ischemia, prerenal azotemia, sepsis, or other nephrotoxins, should always be considered. It is possible, for example, that CIN might be mistaken for cholesterol crystal embolization after intravascular catheterization.

In summary, potential causes of CIN include altered rheologic properties, perturbation of renal hemodynamics, regional hypoxia, auto- and paracrine factors (adenosine, endothelin, reactive oxygen species), and direct cytotoxic effects.

Pathophysiology of CIN

Since the 1950s, triiodobenzene has provided the basis for the various available CM. CM are normally grouped according to their osmolality and ionicity. Early on, high-osmolar CM (having osmolalities approximately 6-fold higher than plasma) were widely used, and the differentiation with regard to osmolality made sense. However, it has become clear that many of the side-effects were caused by the electric charge and currently only low-osmolar CM (which still have a considerably higher osmolality than plasma) and iso-osmolar CM are widely used. Therefore, it appears that the subdivision of CM according to their osmolality may require reconsideration. Iso-osmolar CM are dimers and, correspondingly, reveal greater viscosities than the monomeric low-osmolar CM (Figure 1.1). This can have important implications for renal and systemic hemodynamics, as outlined below.

Although several suggestions have been put forward, the underlying mechanism of CIN remains unclear. Rheologic alterations, activation of the tubuloglomerular feedback (TGF) response, regional hypoxia, cytotoxic effects on the renal epithelial cells, generation of reactive oxygen species, and, finally, increased adenosine or endothelin production are among the possible mechanisms behind CIN that will be outlined here.

Tubular concentration of CM and rheology

The pressure of the vessels supplying the renal medulla with blood is only about 17 mmHg (for review see reference 13). Along the renal tubular system, substances like CM that are not reabsorbed become increasingly concentrated. Up to 99% of renal fluids are usually taken up by the action of manifold cellular and paracellular mechanisms. This means that the concentration of CM can increase by a factor of 100. Along with the continuous concentration process, tubular fluid containing CM will become increasingly viscous and can lead to tubular obstruction. Indeed, tubular pressure of over 40 mmHg has been measured after infusion of high-viscosity (dimeric)

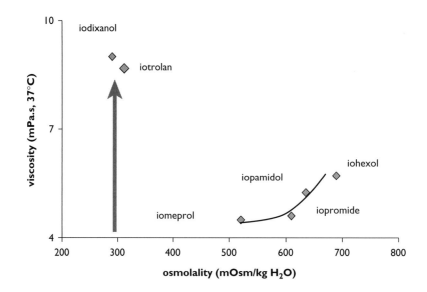

Figure 1.1 *Osmolality and viscosity for I-concentration of 300 mg/ml*

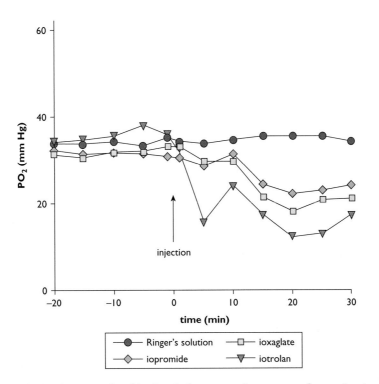

Figure 1.2 *Medullary hypoxia induced by CM. Reduction in pO$_2$ is greatest for iotrolan (iso-osmolar non-ionic dimer) followed by ioxaglate (low-osmolar ionic dimer). Iopromide (low-osmolar monomer) had the least effect on medullary pO$_2$. (From Liss et al,[15] with permission.)*

CM.[14] Inevitably, intrarenal pressure increases as well, since the kidney cannot expand due to the surrounding capsule. As a consequence, renal perfusion pressure for the renal medulla (17 mmHg) may no longer be high enough to warrant sufficient perfusion to critical kidney regions.

There is a relationship between osmolality and viscosity among the monomeric CM (Figure 1.1). However, since iso-osmolar CM exhibit considerably higher viscosity due to their dimeric structure, iso-osmolar CM should impair the renal medullary blood flow to a greater extent than low-osmolar agents. Indeed, this appears to be true, looking at the particularly reduced pO$_2$ levels caused by iso-osmolar CM[15] (Figure 1.2).

The adverse effects of augmented fluid viscosity due to the use of dimeric CM may be more pronounced in the renal tubules than in the capillaries. Since the ultrafiltrate contains very few plasma proteins, it is normal for the tubular fluid to have a lower viscosity than plasma. Using dimeric CM will enhance tubular fluid viscosity, and so increase the resistance to flow in renal tubules.[16] Viscosity is exponentially related to concentration; thus, tubular fluid viscosity increases throughout the passage of the tubular system. Depending upon the hydration status, tubular clotting can occur, particularly when using CM with high viscosity (iodixanol and iotrolan). Urine viscosity following administration of dimeric CM of different viscosities is depicted in Figure 1.3. A scheme of the adverse effects of pronounced increases in viscosity on the kidney is presented in Figure 1.4.

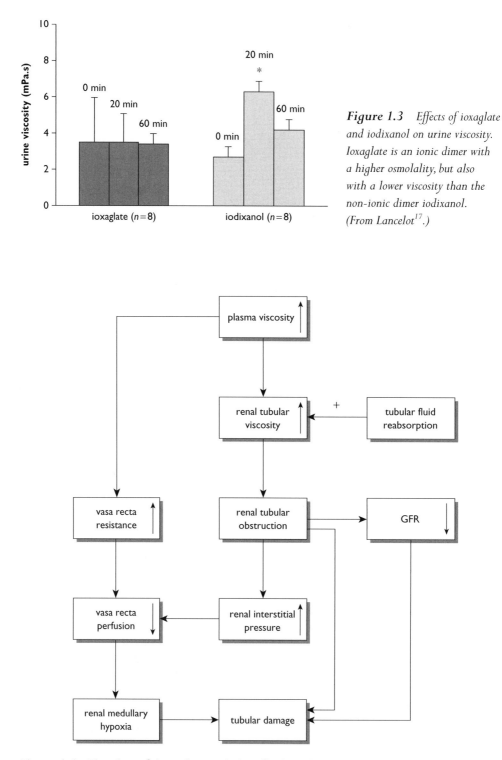

Figure 1.3 *Effects of ioxaglate and iodixanol on urine viscosity. Ioxaglate is an ionic dimer with a higher osmolality, but also with a lower viscosity than the non-ionic dimer iodixanol. (From Lancelot[17].)*

Figure 1.4 *Flow chart of the mechanisms linking fluid osmolality to renal damage.*

The macula densa mechanism

The macula densa mechanism, which is commonly referred to as the TGF, is a powerful and potent mechanism in the control of renal vascular resistance and glomerular filtration. It plays an important role in a popular explanation for the development of CIN: hyperosmotic CM cause diuresis, which activates the TGF and subsequently compromises renal blood flow and glomerular filtration. Nevertheless, this osmotic diuresis theory is not a likely explanation for CIN. The macula densa cells of the thick ascending limb detect Na^+, K^+, and Cl^- concentrations in the tubular fluid via the $Na^+/K^+/2Cl^-$ cotransporter. This transporter is effectively blocked by furosemide. The affinity for Cl^- is very low, so in a physiologic setting there will always be enough Na^+ and K^+ to keep the system running, and Cl^- is the limiting factor.[18,19] Pioneering experiments with retrograde perfusions of the tubule have already shown that osmolality has no effect on the TGF.

Experiments using mannitol together with an osmotic diuretic further support the elimination of the osmotic diuresis theory. Increases in osmolality, such as after mannitol infusion or after CM application, decrease NaCl concentration at the macula densa, while simultaneously increasing tubular flow. Therefore, the resulting net change in the amount of NaCl passing the macula densa is negligible.[20] It is important to note that blocking the TGF by furosemide does not decrease serum creatinine after application of CM, which is usually the parameter taken to indicate CIN.[2] Combining this evidence negates the likelihood that the osmolality of a contrast medium causes CIN via the TGF.

Regional hypoxia

Kidney perfusion is extremely high for the cortex, but the medullary portions are maintained at the verge of hypoxia where pO_2 levels can be as low as 20 mmHg.[21] Such is the consequence of upholding the countercurrent mechanism for controlling urine excretion. The deeper portion of the outer medulla is a particularly vulnerable kidney region. It is an area remote from the vasa recta, that supplies the renal medulla with blood (Figure 1.5). This is where the thick ascending limbs of the loop of Henle exhibit hypoxic damage, for example when the kidney is perfused with erythrocyte-free medium.[22] The relatively high oxygen requirements due to salt reabsorption account for the vulnerability of the outer medullary portion of the nephron. By increasing renal vascular resistance, the addition of CM to the medium probably aggravates hypoxic injury to this region.[23] It has been reported that an iso-osmolar contrast medium, iodixanol (a dimer with high viscosity), reduces blood flow to all regions of the kidney to a greater extent than low-osmolar, and even high-osmolar CM. However, this decrease in perfusion was more likely due to profound systemic effects of iodixanol, since blood pressure also dropped considerably.[24] In a later study in dogs with stable blood pressure, the greater risk of high-viscosity CM for inducing renal medullary hypoxia was indeed documented (Figure 1.6).[17]

Iothalamate, a high-osmolar agent, markedly reduces medullary pO_2 to about a third of control levels.[25] Strikingly, the iso-osmolar CM iotrolan impairs local pO_2 to a greater extent than the low-osmolar CM iopromide.[26] In fact, the decrease in pO_2 by the latter failed to reach statistical significance (Figure 1.2). These results underscore the shortcoming of classifying CM simply by their osmolality.

Some systemic effects of CM, such as transiently reduced cardiac output[27] and a suboptimal pulmonary perfusion–ventilation relationship,[28] can aggravate local renal hypoxia. Additionally, since CM can increase oxygen affinity of hemoglobin, oxygen delivery to the peripheral tissues may be attenuated.[29]

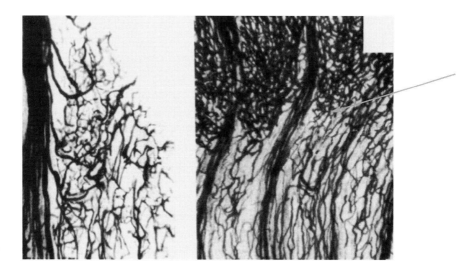

Figure 1.5 *Injection study of vascular bundles in the outer medulla (OM) of the rat (left and right). Individual vascular bundles are more evenly dispersed throughout the inner stripe of the OM. This pattern is most typical of mammalian species including the rat, mouse, and human. The area at risk of CIN is the inner stripe of the outer medulla (arrow), where the vascular density decrease. (From Pallone et al,[13] with permission.)*

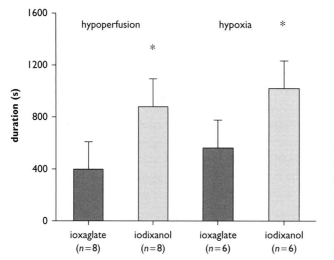

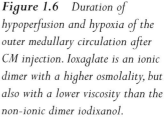

Figure 1.6 *Duration of hypoperfusion and hypoxia of the outer medullary circulation after CM injection. Ioxaglate is an ionic dimer with a higher osmolality, but also with a lower viscosity than the non-ionic dimer iodixanol.*

Blocking the transporters in this nephron segment should have beneficial effects on the prevention of CIN, if renal outer medullary hypoxia causes CIN. The bulk of transport taking place in the medullary thick ascending limb is the $Na^+/K^+/2Cl^-$ transporter, which, as mentioned above, is blocked by furosemide. If the transport were blocked, it would dramatically lower local oxygen consumption and alleviate the reduced oxygen supply. In fact, this has been demonstrated in

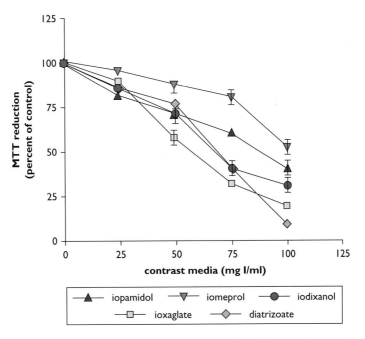

Figure 1.7 *Altered mitochondrial function in a proximal tubular cell line as determined by 3-(4,5-dimethylthiazol-2-yl)-2,5-diphenyltetrazolium bromide (MTT) reduction (24-hour treatment). A comparison of the effects of various CM on MTT reduction reveals significant differences from one another (P < 0.01). The least influence was found by the low-osmolar agents, followed by the iso-osmolar CM (iodixanol). The ionic substances showed the greatest effect. (From Hardiek et al,[31] with permission.)*

experiments in rats, showing that outer medullary pO_2 is elevated after furosemide.[30] Nevertheless, CM injection after furosemide still reduces outer medullary pO_2, although it occurs at higher absolute pO_2 values. Interestingly, furosemide given just before angiography fails to limit increases in serum creatinine after CM application, implying that yet other mechanisms are involved in CIN.[2]

Cytotoxic effects on renal tubular (epithelial) cells

In vitro investigations on cell lines are routinely used for assessing renal tubular cell function or damage. A porcine proximal tubular cell line, LLC-PK1, was used by Hardiek et al[31] to investigate CIN. Although proliferation was impaired, an effect on apoptosis was not found. Reduced proliferation will affect renal function but with a delay of hours or days, which may help explain the clinical course of CIN. Regardless of the CM used, tubular cell uptake can occur as indicated by vacuolization.[32] A more explicit indicator of proximal tubular function seems to be a perturbation of mitochondrial enzyme activity and mitochondrial membrane potential[31] (Figure 1.7). The extent of mitochondrial enzyme activity impairment relies primarily on two features of the CM: ionicity and the molecular structure. Notably, low-osmolar (monomeric) CM had the least effect, followed by the iso-osmolar (dimeric, non-ionic) agents. As expected, ionic compounds revealed the most profound effects.[31] In the distal tubule, CM may promote apoptosis, as indicated in the MDCK cell line model.[33] This partly seems to rely on hypoxic damage;[34] however, there is also a direct influence on these cells.[33] CM can also open the intercellular junctions and affect the polarity of the epithelial cell surface.[35] These features are important for normal fluid and electrolyte reabsorption and may add to the potential deleterious effects of CM.

Reactive oxygen species (ROS), adenosine and endothelin

Even under normal conditions, oxygen radicals are produced endogenously, but oxidative stress exacerbates the levels. Among the most common oxygen radicals are superoxide (O_2^-), hydrogen peroxide (H_2O_2), and hydroxyl radical (OH^-).[36] Superoxide and hydroxyl radicals are more reactive than H_2O_2, which is not a radical, but exhibits greater membrane permeability.

Endothelial dysfunction in renal vessels is a common sequela in diabetes mellitus, one of the most prominent risk factors for CIN. It appears that the tonic influence of NO in the renal microvasculature is suppressed and contributes to the endothelial dysfunction in the early stages of insulin-dependent diabetes.[36] The attenuated NO activity in the diabetic renal microvasculature can be explained: the superoxide rapidly scavenges NO. Supporting this hypothesis, superoxide production was found to be increased in renal cortical tissue from diabetic rats.[37] Moreover, Ohishi and Carmines[38] demonstrated that for juxtamedullary nephrons of streptozotocin-diabetic rats, the afferent and efferent arteriolar vasoconstrictor response to NOS inhibition is impaired. Additionally, a recent study by Palm and coworkers[39] showed that scavenger treatment (vitamin E) normalizes the reduced pO_2 found in the renal medulla of streptozotocin-diabetic rats. With the understanding that NO inhibits oxygen consumption, it is tempting to speculate that reduced (scavenged) NO during diabetes elevates oxygen consumption. This would lead to reduced pO_2 with consequences for endothelial–epithelial structure and function.

Interestingly, ROS may play a role in the effects of various vasoconstrictors that have been considered important for the development of CIN. Since ROS are extracellular signaling molecules, they are potentially significant in mediating the actions of vasoconstrictors, such as angiotensin II, TXA_2, endothelin-1, adenosine, and norepinephrine. Moreover, various models of renal inflammation and ischemia have displayed a role of ROS in glomerular injury. It is possible, then, that the adverse effects of CM on renal function may involve the generation of ROS, for example via adenosine formation. This notion is supported by experiments in which the generation of ROS was inhibited by allopurinol and experiments where the amount of ROS was reduced by superoxide dismutase. In these models, CM-induced reductions in glomerular filtration rate are attenuated.[40] Later additional studies performed in humans further underscore a role for ROS in CIN.[41]

Considering the strong evidence supporting a role for ROS in CIN, it is not surprising that clinical trials have been performed with the aim of ameliorating CIN by scavenging ROS.[42–45] In these trials, N-acetylcysteine was given in addition to the general hydration protocols and showed a positive outcome in four of the studies.[42,43,45,46] N-Acetylcysteine administration has therefore been recommended for the prevention of CIN in patients with mild-to-moderate renal insufficiency.[47] However, it must be made clear that this recommendation is not unequivocal.[48]

Adenosine in the kidney exerts a vasoconstrictor response on the afferent arteriole, due to the predominance of A_1 receptors.[49] Early studies indicated the existence of both A_1 and A_{2A} receptors in the kidney. They were found to be widely distributed throughout the renal vasculature, juxtaglomerular apparatus, glomeruli, tubules, and collecting ducts.[50,51] In addition to its vasoconstrictor effect, A_1 receptor stimulation contracts mesangial cells in the glomerulus.[52] In 1982, Osswald and colleagues[53] proposed that metabolic demand controls kidney hemodynamics, and suggested adenosine as the mediator of the TGF due to its particular vasoconstrictor response in renal circulation. Since then, this hypothesis has been considerably substantiated by experiments demonstrating lacking TGF responses in mice devoid of adenosine A_1 receptors.[54–56]

Due to the prominent role of adenosine in the renal vascular bed, several studies have targeted the role of adenosine in CIN.[57–59] In diabetes mellitus, an even higher sensitivity of the renal vasculature to adenosine is found, suggesting that adenosine is an important contributor to CIN in patients suffering from this metabolic disorder.[60] In spite of adenosine's strategic role in renal function, the part it plays in CIN appears to be overestimated. The adenosine A_1 receptor is not involved in the depression of outer medullary blood flow and oxygen tension caused by injection of CM, as shown in a recent study in a normal rat.[61] In that study, a specific A_1 receptor antagonist was administered together with CM. Although a pronounced basal influence of A_1 receptors on renal medullary hemodynamics was confirmed, the resulting blocking of these receptors failed to alleviate medullary hypoperfusion and hypoxia in response to the CM. The general reduction in renal plasma flow and GFR by CM is not attributable to enhanced adenosine action,[57] and further supports the limited role of adenosine in CIN.

The effects of endothelin on vascular beds primarily depend on the receptor subtype activation. ET-A receptor stimulation elicits pronounced vasoconstriction, whereas the ET-B receptor has the opposite effect. Most likely, the latter involves endothelin-dependent NO release. Recently, however, both subtypes of receptors were found to mediate the vasoconstrictor action of endothelins in human blood vessels.[62] The net vasoactive response to endothelin is believed to vary depending on the vascular bed in question.

The association of endothelin with CIN appears likely due to the enhanced endothelin levels in plasma and urine, which are observed after radiocontrast administration.[63–65] Additionally, it is known that the transcription and release of endothelin from endothelial cells is enhanced by CM (for review see reference 66). Moreover, patients suffering from impaired renal function evince an exaggerated increase in endothelin after receiving CM.[67] However, the aggregate effect of endothelin in the scenario of CIN may not be as disadvantageous as one may assume from the findings mentioned above. As the study by Wang et al showed,[68] when both ET-A and ET-B receptors are blocked in humans receiving CM, the mean increase in serum creatinine concentration is significantly greater in patients receiving the ET-A/ET-B blocker compared to those who received placebo. Moreover, the CIN incidence is significantly higher in patients who receive this blocker compared to placebo.

A potentially advantageous result of endothelin in the development of CIN may be explained by the ET-B-mediated effects, for example vasodilatation. Accordingly, a selective ET-A receptor blockade could prove to be serviceable in the prevention of CIN. In the study of Wang et al,[68] when the unselective blocker was used, plasma endothelin-1 levels may have increased, as shown by a study employing a similar iv infusion of the same endothelin receptor antagonist, SB 209670.[69] This increase in endothelin-1 concentration is probably accomplished by the ET-B receptor antagonism,[70] since one of the ET-B-mediated effects is the attenuation of further endothelin release. Thus, the potentiation of CIN induced by SB 209670 in the study of Wang et al. could be explained by ET-B receptor blockade increasing plasma endothelin, which then acts on the ET-A receptor.[71] Indeed, studies in the normal rat have reported a positive effect of ET-A-selective blockade on the renal outer medullary hypoxic response to CM.[72] Remarkably, the hypoxia in this kidney region was alleviated without enhancing local blood flow. Hence, it was concluded that the oxygen requirements must have decreased due to ET-A antagonism. This, in fact, may be an important clue for understanding the role of endothelin in CIN. It appears that BQ123, a selective ET-A antagonist, inhibits Na^+/K^+-ATPase activity.[53,72] If this were to occur in the kidneys, a reduction in oxygen demand in the outer medulla would be readily explainable.

The issue of osmolality: functional considerations and clinical studies

The use of the more modern CM that are low- or iso-osmolar has reduced the likelihood of CIN occurrence, in comparison to high-osmolar CM. In a prospective, randomized study involving 1196 low-risk patients (patients without diabetes who had a base-line serum creatinine concentration of less than 1.5 mg/dl [133 μmol/l], Rudnick et al[4] discovered no differences in the incidence of nephropathy between patients receiving iohexol (low-osmolar; 780 mOsm/kg H_2O) and those receiving diatrizoate (high-osmolar; 1870 mOsm/kg H_2O). However, in patients without diabetes, whose serum creatinine concentrations were higher than 1.5 mg/dl, the incidence of nephropathy was reduced from 27.0 to 12.2% by the use of iohexol.[4] For patients with diabetes, the incidence was reduced from 47.7 to 33.3%. In total, patients receiving high-osmolar CM were 3.3 times as likely to develop CIN as those receiving low-osmolar CM. For all practical purposes, all the newer low-osmolar or iso-osmolar agents were considered to be the preferred agents in patients at higher than usual risk for the development of CIN.[9]

Additional comparative studies in patients with pre-existing renal impairment have shown similar susceptibility for CIN in both non-ionic monomeric and non-ionic dimeric CM,[73–75] whereas other trials have concluded that iso-osmolar CM have advantages with regard to the occurrence of CIN in renal impaired patients.[1,76] In particular, Aspelin et al, in the NEPHRIC study, concluded that iohexol ($n = 65$) was significantly more nephrotoxic than the non-ionic dimer iodixanol ($n = 64$) in patients with pre-existing chronic renal failure and diabetes undergoing coronary or aortofemoral angiography.[1] The conclusions of the authors have exposed these results to considerable attention; however, some shortcomings of the study design have also raised some comment. Previous studies have shown that critical determinants for the susceptibility of CIN are duration of diabetes, metabolic status, and renal function before CM injection.[7] These factors prove particularly important when interpreting the patient groups investigated in the study of Aspelin and coworkers, since they were significantly different in the study. With this in mind, the outcome of the study is likely also to reflect the differences of the studied populations rather than differences of the administered CM with regard to CIN. An additional negator lies in the fact that a uniform hydration regimen was not pursued with vigor, as indicated by the considerable variance in fluid intake.

The conclusion of the NEPHRIC study that the use of iso-osmolar CM, as opposed to low-osmolar CM, results in reduced incidence of CIN is not fully in line with our current understanding of CIN, as mentioned above, and contradicts studies in which the use of iso-osmolar CM confers no advantage.[24,77] In the light of the controversy as to whether patients at risk actually benefit from iso-osmolar CM[1,76] or not,[73–75] and the experimental data on physiologic/pathophysiologic renal mechanisms that do not support any beneficial effects of iso-osmolar CM, the CM of choice still remains an open question.[78]

Pathophysiology in the prevention of CIN by hydration

Unfortunately, an open question remains the treatment strategies to prevent CIN, which have yet to be established. Several proposals for CIN prevention have been reported, of which vigorous hydration may be the most important.[79,80] Currently, only periprocedural hydration is widely accepted to prevent CIN[2,81,82] and intravenous hydration tests better than oral hydration. The reason for the success of hydration is not related to an increase in renal blood flow or glomerular filtration rate (as sometimes thought).[83] Unless the patient is severely dehydrated, volume loading has little effect on these hemodynamic measures. It appears more likely that medullary perfusion is increased when the patient is well hydrated. Autoregulation may not be present under these conditions[84] and suppressed vasopressin levels augment medullary blood flow;[85,86] thus, regional pO_2 is enhanced.

Furthermore, and perhaps more importantly, the CM concentration in the tubular system is reduced when the patient is hydrated. Volume expansion and decreases in plasma osmolality prevent re-uptake of water in the collecting ducts. This occurs by inhibition of arginine vasopressin (AVP) via vagal inputs from the mechanoreceptors located at the atrial–venous junctions and by a direct effect of osmolality on the supraoptic nuclei. In consequence, fewer aquaporins are inserted into the wall of the collecting duct cells. Thus, water remains in the collecting ducts and the CM become less concentrated. This dilution process decreases the viscosity of the collecting duct fluid and facilitates CM excretion. If the patient is volume depleted, the concentration of CM in the collecting duct is significantly increased, theoretically by a factor of up to 100-fold greater than that in the plasma. This increases tubular pressure and intrarenal tissue pressure. The latter causes damage by decreasing blood flow to the renal medulla.

Conclusions

There may not be a single cause for CIN. Several pathophysiologic mechanisms can add up to impair kidney function. The use of newer CM and extracellular fluid volume expansion are to be preferred in patients with pre-existing renal impairments.[2,79,87]

With regard to the current concepts to explain CIN, the rheologic properties of a fluid may not have received sufficient attention. Resistance depends on fluid viscosity, not osmolality (Poiseuille's law). Moreover, osmolality does not directly affect the TGF, as already shown by the pioneer work in this field.[18,19] Thus, perhaps too much attention has been directed to the osmolality of different CM, while neglecting the impact of other physicochemic properties. Indeed, there is little experimental evidence that would support the notion that iso-osmolar CM are superior to the low-osmolar agents in preventing CIN. In fact, the contrary has been demonstrated. Further studies comparing iso- with low-osmolar CM in patients at risk are required before any conclusions can be drawn as to the possible superiority of certain CM. In these awaited studies, the importance of well-controlled and sufficient hydration status cannot be overestimated.

References

1. Aspelin P, Aubry P, Fransson SG et al. Nephrotoxic effects in high-risk patients undergoing angiography. *N Engl J Med* 2003; **348**:491–9.

2. Solomon R, Werner C, Mann D, D'Elia J, Silva P. Effects of saline, mannitol, and furosemide to prevent acute decreases in renal function induced by radiocontrast agents. *N Engl J Med* 1994; **331**:1416–20.

3. Barrett BJ, Parfrey PS, Vavasour HM et al. Contrast nephropathy in patients with impaired renal function: high versus low osmolar media. *Kidney Int* 1992; **41**:1274–9.

4. Rudnick MR, Goldfarb S, Wexler L et al. Nephrotoxicity of ionic and nonionic contrast media in 1196 patients: a randomized trial. The Iohexol Cooperative Study. *Kidney Int* 1995; **47**:254–61.

5. Taliercio CP, Vlietstra RE, Ilstrup DM et al. A randomized comparison of the nephrotoxicity of iopamidol and diatrizoate in high risk patients undergoing cardiac angiography. *J Am Coll Cardiol* 1991; **17**:384–90.

6. Manske CL, Sprafka JM, Strony JT, Wang Y. Contrast nephropathy in azotemic diabetic patients undergoing coronary angiography. *Am J Med* 1990; **89**:615–20.

7. Waybill MM, Waybill PN. Contrast media-induced nephrotoxicity: identification of patients at risk and algorithms for prevention. *J Vasc Interv Radiol* 2001; **12**:3–9.

8. Levy EM, Viscoli CM, Horwitz RI. The effect of acute renal failure on mortality. A cohort analysis. *JAMA* 1996; **275**:1489–94.

9. Thomsen HS, Morcos SK. Contrast media and the kidney: European Society of Urogenital Radiology (ESUR) guidelines. *Br J Radiol* 2003; **76**:513–18.

10. Parfrey PS, Griffiths SM, Barrett BJ et al. Contrast material-induced renal failure in patients with diabetes mellitus, renal insufficiency, or both. A prospective controlled study. *N Engl J Med* 1989; **320**:143–9.

11. Berns AS. Nephrotoxicity of contrast media. *Kidney Int* 1989; **36**:730–40.

12. Deray G, Cacoub P, Jacquiaud C et al. Renal tolerance for ioxaglate in patients with chronic renal failure. *Radiology* 1991; **179**:395–7.

13. Pallone TL, Turner MR, Edwards A, Jamison RL. Countercurrent exchange in the renal medulla. *Am J Physiol Regul Integr Comp Physiol* 2003; **284**:R1153–R1175.

14. Ueda J, Nygren A, Hansell P, Ulfendahl HR. Effect of intravenous contrast media on proximal and distal tubular hydrostatic pressure in the rat kidney. *Acta Radiol* 1993; **34**:83–7.

15. Liss P, Nygren A, Erikson U, Ulfendahl HR. Injection of low and iso-osmolar contrast medium decreases oxygen tension in the renal medulla. *Kidney Int* 1998; **53**:698–702.

16. Ueda J, Nygren A, Hansell P, Erikson U. Influence of contrast media on single nephron glomerular filtration rate in rat kidney. A comparison between diatrizoate, iohexol, ioxaglate, and iotrolan. *Acta Radiol* 1992; **33**:596–9.

17. Lancelot E, Idee JM, Lacledere C et al. Effects of two dimeric iodinated contrast media on renal medullary blood perfusion and oxygenation in dogs. *Invest Radiol* 2002; **37**:368–75.

18. Schnermann J, Ploth DW, Hermle M. Activation of tubulo-glomerular feedback by chloride transport. *Pflugers Arch* 1976; **362**:229–40.

19. Briggs JP, Schnermann J, Wright FS. Failure of tubule fluid osmolarity to affect feedback regulation of glomerular filtration. *Am J Physiol* 1980; **239**:F427–F432.

20. Leyssac PP, Holstein-Rathlou NH, Skott O. Renal blood flow, early distal sodium, and plasma renin concentrations during osmotic diuresis. *Am J Physiol Regul Integr Comp Physiol* 2000; **279**:R1268–R1276.

21. Brezis M, Rosen S. Hypoxia of the renal medulla – its implications for disease. *N Engl J Med* 1995; **332**:647–55.

22. Brezis M, Rosen S, Silva P, Epstein FH. Selective vulnerability of the medullary thick ascending limb to anoxia in the isolated perfused rat kidney. *J Clin Invest* 1984; **73**:182–90.

23. Heyman SN, Brezis M, Reubinoff CA et al. Acute renal failure with selective medullary injury in the rat. *J Clin Invest* 1988; **82**:401–12.

24. Lancelot E, Idee JM, Couturier V, Vazin V, Corot C. Influence of the viscosity of iodixanol on medullary and cortical blood flow in the rat kidney: a potential cause of nephrotoxicity. *J Appl Toxicol* 1999; **19**:341–6.

25. Heyman SN, Reichman J, Brezis M. Pathophysiology of radiocontrast nephropathy: a role for medullary hypoxia. *Invest Radiol* 1999; **34**:685–91.

26. Liss P, Nygren A, Erikson U, Ulfendahl HR. Injection of low and iso-osmolar contrast medium decreases oxygen tension in the renal medulla. *Kidney Int* 1998; **53**:698–702.

27. Dawson P. Cardiovascular effects of contrast agents. *Am J Cardiol* 1989; **64**:2E–9E.

28. Neagley SR, Vought MB, Weidner WA, Zwillich CW. Transient oxygen desaturation following radiographic contrast medium administration. *Arch Intern Med* 1986; **146**:1094–7.

29. Kim SJ, Salem MR, Joseph NJ et al. Contrast media adversely affect oxyhemoglobin dissociation. *Anesth Analg* 1990; **71**:73–6.

30. Liss P, Nygren A, Ulfendahl HR, Erikson U. Effect of furosemide or mannitol before injection of a non-ionic contrast medium on intrarenal oxygen tension. *Adv Exp Med Biol* 1999; **471**:353–9.

31. Hardiek K, Katholi RE, Ramkumar V, Deitrick C. Proximal tubule cell response to radiographic contrast media. *Am J Physiol Renal Physiol* 2001; **280**:F61–F70.

32. Andersen KJ, Christensen EI, Vik H. Effects of iodinated x-ray contrast media on renal epithelial cells in culture. *Invest Radiol* 1994; **29**:955–62.

33. Hizoh I, Strater J, Schick CS, Kubler W, Haller C. Radiocontrast-induced DNA fragmentation of renal tubular cells in vitro: role of hypertonicity. *Nephrol Dial Transplant* 1998; **13**:911–18.

34. Beeri R, Symon Z, Brezis M et al. Rapid DNA fragmentation from hypoxia along the thick ascending limb of rat kidneys. *Kidney Int* 1995; **47**:1806–10.

35. Haller C, Schick CS, Zorn M, Kubler W. Cytotoxicity of radiocontrast agents on polarized renal epithelial cell monolayers. *Cardiovasc Res* 1997; **33**:655–65.

36. Schnackenberg CG. Physiological and pathophysiological roles of oxygen radicals in the renal microvasculature. *Am J Physiol Regul Integr Comp Physiol* 2002; **282**:R335–R342.

37. Ishii N, Patel KP, Lane PH et al. Nitric oxide synthesis and oxidative stress in the renal cortex of rats with diabetes mellitus. *J Am Soc Nephrol* 2001; **12**:1630–9.

38. Ohishi K, Carmines PK. Superoxide dismutase restores the influence of nitric oxide on renal arterioles in diabetes mellitus. *J Am Soc Nephrol* 1995; **5**:1559–66.

39. Palm F, Cederberg J, Hansell P, Liss P, Carlsson PO. Reactive oxygen species cause diabetes-induced decrease in renal oxygen tension. *Diabetologia* 2003; **46**:1153–60.

40. Bakris GL, Lass N, Gaber AO, Jones JD, Burnett JC Jr. Radiocontrast medium-induced declines in renal function: a role for oxygen free radicals. *Am J Physiol* 1990; **258(1 Pt 2)**:F115–F120.

41. Katholi RE, Woods WT Jr, Taylor GJ et al. Oxygen free radicals and contrast nephropathy. *Am J Kidney Dis* 1998; **32**:64–71.

42. Tepel M, van der Giet M, Schwarzfeld C et al. Prevention of radiographic-contrast-agent-induced reductions in renal function by acetylcysteine. *N Engl J Med* 2000; **343**:180–4.

43. Diaz-Sandoval LJ, Kosowsky BD, Losordo DW. Acetylcysteine to prevent angiography-related renal tissue injury (the APART trial). *Am J Cardiol* 2002; **89**:356–8.

44. Briguori C, Manganelli F, Scarpato P et al. Acetylcysteine and contrast agent-associated nephrotoxicity. *J Am Coll Cardiol* 2002; **40**:298–303.

45. Shyu KG, Cheng JJ, Kuan P. Acetylcysteine protects against acute renal damage in patients with abnormal renal function undergoing a coronary procedure. *J Am Coll Cardiol* 2002; **40**:1383–8.

46. Kay J, Chow WH, Chan TM et al. Acetylcysteine for prevention of acute deterioration of renal function following elective coronary angiography and intervention: a randomized controlled trial. *JAMA* 2003; **289**:553–8.

47. Walker PD, Brokering KL, Theobald JC. Fenoldopam and *N*-acetylcysteine for the prevention of radiographic contrast material-induced nephropathy: a review. *Pharmacotherapy* 2003; **23**:1617–26.

48. Durham JD, Caputo C, Dokko J et al. A randomized controlled trial of *N*-acetylcysteine to prevent contrast nephropathy in cardiac angiography. *Kidney Int* 2002; **62**:2202–7.

49. Weihprecht H, Lorenz JN, Briggs JP, Schnermann J. Vasomotor effects of purinergic agonists in isolated rabbit afferent arterioles. *Am J Physiol* 1992; **263(6 Pt 2)**:F1026–F1033.

50. Weaver DR, Reppert SM. Adenosine receptor gene expression in rat kidney. *Am J Physiol* 1992; **263 (6 Pt 2)**:F991–F995.

51. Spielman WS, Arend LJ. Adenosine receptors and signaling in the kidney. *Hypertension* 1991; **17**:117–30.

52. Olivera A, Lamas S, Rodriguez-Puyol D, Lopez-Novoa JM. Adenosine induces mesangial cell contraction by an A1-type receptor. *Kidney Int* 1989; **35**:1300–5.

53. Osswald H, Hermes HH, Nabakowski G. Role of adenosine in signal transmission of tubuloglomerular feedback. *Kidney Int Suppl* 1982; **12**:S136–S142.

54. Sun D, Samuelson LC, Yang T et al. Mediation of tubuloglomerular feedback by adenosine: evidence from mice lacking adenosine 1 receptors. *Proc Natl Acad Sci USA* 2001; **98**:9983–8.

55. Brown R, Ollerstam A, Johansson B et al. Abolished tubuloglomerular feedback and increased plasma renin in adenosine A1 receptor-deficient mice. *Am J Physiol Regul Integr Comp Physiol* 2001; **281**: R1362–R1367.

56. Persson PB. Tubuloglomerular feedback in adenosine A1 receptor-deficient mice. *Am J Physiol Regul Integr Comp Physiol* 2001; **281**:R1361.

57. Oldroyd SD, Fang L, Haylor JL et al. Effects of adenosine receptor antagonists on the responses to contrast media in the isolated rat kidney. *Clin Sci (Lond)* 2000; **98**:303–11.

58. Katholi RE, Taylor GJ, McCann WP et al. Nephrotoxicity from contrast media: attenuation with theophylline. *Radiology* 1995; **195**:17-22.

59. Arakawa K, Suzuki H, Naitoh M et al. Role of adenosine in the renal responses to contrast medium. *Kidney Int* 1996; **49**:1199–206.

60. Pflueger A, Larson TS, Nath KA et al. Role of adenosine in contrast media-induced acute renal failure in diabetes mellitus. *Mayo Clin Proc* 2000; **75**:1275–83.

61. Liss P, Carlsson PO, Palm F, Hansell P. Adenosine A(1) receptors in contrast media-induced renal dysfunction in the normal rat. *Eur Radiol* 2004; **14**:1297–302.

62. Seo B, Oemar BS, Siebenmann R, von Segesser L, Luscher TF. Both ETA and ETB receptors mediate contraction to endothelin-1 in human blood vessels. *Circulation* 1994; **89**:1203–8.

63. Bagnis C, Idee JM, Dubois M et al. Role of endothelium-derived nitric oxide–endothelin balance in contrast medium-induced acute renal vasoconstriction in dogs. *Acad Radiol* 1997; **4**:343–8.

64. Clark BA, Kim D, Epstein FH. Endothelin and atrial natriuretic peptide levels following radiocontrast exposure in humans. *Am J Kidney Dis* 1997; **30**:82–6.

65. Heyman SN, Clark BA, Kaiser N et al. Radiocontrast agents induce endothelin release in vivo and in vitro. *J Am Soc Nephrol* 1992; **3**:58–65.

66. Oldroyd SD, Morcos SK. Endothelin: what does the radiologist need to know? *Br J Radiol* 2000; **73**:1246–51.

67. Fujisaki K, Kubo M, Masuda K et al. Infusion of radiocontrast agents induces exaggerated release of urinary endothelin in patients with impaired renal function. *Clin Exp Nephrol* 2003; **7**:279–83.

68. Wang A, Holcslaw T, Bashore TM et al. Exacerbation of radiocontrast nephrotoxicity by endothelin receptor antagonism. *Kidney Int* 2000; **57**:1675–80.

69. Freed MI, Wilson DE, Thompson KA et al. Pharmacokinetics and pharmacodynamics of SB 209670, an endothelin receptor antagonist: effects on the regulation of renal vascular tone. *Clin Pharmacol Ther* 1999; **65**:473–82.

70. Weber C, Schmitt R, Birnboeck H et al. Pharmacokinetics and pharmacodynamics of the endothelin-receptor antagonist bosentan in healthy human subjects. *Clin Pharmacol Ther* 1996; **60**:124–37.

71. Haylor JL, Morcos SK. An oral ET(A)-selective endothelin receptor antagonist for contrast nephropathy? *Nephrol Dial Transplant* 2001; **16**:1336–7.

72. Liss P, Carlsson PO, Nygren A, Palm F, Hansell P. Et-A receptor antagonist BQ123 prevents radio-contrast media-induced renal medullary hypoxia. *Acta Radiol* 2003; **44**:111–17.

73. Jakobsen JA. Renal experience with Visipaque. *Eur Radiol* 1996; **6(Suppl 2)**:S16–S19.

74. Carraro M, Malalan F, Antonione R et al. Effects of a dimeric vs a monomeric nonionic contrast medium on renal function in patients with mild to moderate renal insufficiency: a double-blind, randomized clinical trial. *Eur Radiol* 1998; **8**:144–7.

75. Andrew E, Berg KJ, Nossen JO et al. Renal effects of iodixanol in patients: a comparison with other radiographic contrast media. *Acad Radiol* 1996; **3(Suppl 2)**:S440–S443.

76. Chalmers N, Jackson RW. Comparison of iodixanol and iohexol in renal impairment. *Br J Radiol* 1999; **72**:701–3.

77. Deray G, Bagnis C, Jacquiaud C et al. Renal effects of low and isoosmolar contrast media on renal hemodynamic in a normal and ischemic dog kidney. *Invest Radiol* 1999; **34**:1–4.

78. Sandler CM. Contrast-agent-induced acute renal dysfunction – is iodixanol the answer? *N Engl J Med* 2003; **348**:551–3.

79. Morcos SK, Thomsen HS, Webb JA. Contrast-media-induced nephrotoxicity: a consensus report. Contrast Media Safety Committee, European Society of Urogenital Radiology (ESUR). *Eur Radiol* 1999; **9**:1602–13.

80. Katzberg RW. Urography into the 21st century: new contrast media, renal handling, imaging characteristics, and nephrotoxicity. *Radiology* 1997; **204**:297–312.

81. Murphy SW, Barrett BJ, Parfrey PS. Contrast nephropathy. *J Am Soc Nephrol* 2000; **11**:177–82.

82. Trivedi HS, Moore H, Nasr S et al. A randomized prospective trial to assess the role of saline hydration on the development of contrast nephrotoxicity. *Nephron Clin Pract* 2003; **93**:C29–C34.

83. Gami AS, Garovic VD. Contrast nephropathy after coronary angiography. *Mayo Clin Proc* 2004; **79**:211–19.

84. Nafz B, Berger K, Rosler C, Persson PB. Kinins modulate the sodium-dependent autoregulation of renal medullary blood flow. *Cardiovasc Res* 1998; **40**:573–9.

85. Franchini KG, Cowley AW Jr. Sensitivity of the renal medullary circulation to plasma vasopressin. *Am J Physiol* 1996; **271(3 Pt 2)**:R647–R653.

86. Franchini KG, Cowley AW Jr. Renal cortical and medullary blood flow responses during water restriction: role of vasopressin. *Am J Physiol* 1996; **270(6 Pt 2)**:R1257–R1264.

87. Thomsen HS, Morcos SK. Radiographic contrast media. *BJU Int* 2000; **86(Suppl 1)**:1–10.

2. EPIDEMIOLOGY AND PREDICTORS OF CONTRAST-INDUCED NEPHROPATHY

Peter A McCullough and Sandeep S Soman

Historical perspective

Evidence that radiocontrast causes nephrotoxicity was first reported in the medical literature in the 1960s.[1,2] Contrast-induced nephropathy (CIN) as a leading cause of acute renal failure was described with increasing frequency over the next 10 to 15 years, largely due to increasing use of radiocontrast studies in patients who were older and sicker, with attendant comorbidities such as diabetes mellitus, renal failure, cardiac failure, and volume depletion (Figure 2.1).[3,4] CIN is currently described as the third commonest cause of hospital-acquired renal failure, accounting for approximately 11% of cases.[5] The incidence of CIN reported in the literature has ranged between 1% and 45%, largely depending on the comorbidities of the study population and parameters used to define CIN.[6]

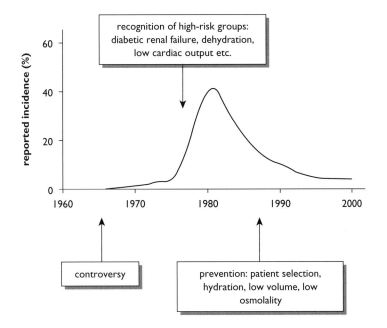

Figure 2.1   *Schematized history of radiocontrast nephropathy. (From Heyman SN, Rosen S, Brezis M.[3], with permission.)*

With more than a million radiocontrast procedures performed annually in the United States, the incidence of CIN is approximately 150 000 cases per year. At least 1% of these episodes require dialysis therapy with prolongation of hospital stay to an average of 17 days, with an additional cost of approximately $32 million annually. For episodes that do not require dialysis, prolongation of the hospital stay by 2 days (at $500 per day) would translate into an added cost of $148 million annually.[7,8] The incidence and costs are higher in critically ill patients with their associated comorbidities, such as hypotension, hypovolemia, diabetes, and congestive heart failure.

Cardiorenal disease

The modern day, first world epidemics of obesity and hypertension are central drivers of a secondary epidemic of combined chronic kidney disease (CKD) and cardiovascular disease (CVD).[9] Approximately half of those with diabetes will develop diabetic nephropathy. Conversely, half of all cases of endstage renal disease (ESRD) are due to diabetic nephropathy.[10] With the graying of America, and cardiovascular care shifting towards the elderly, there is an imperative to understand why decreasing levels of renal dysfunction act as a major adverse prognostic factor after contrast exposure with or without peripheral or percutaneous coronary intervention (PCI). Acute renal failure (ARF) as the most proximal renal event is predictable, and highlights an opportunity for preventive measures which are outlined in this chapter.

Small rises in creatinine are linked to poor long-term outcomes

We and others have demonstrated that the overall risk of CIN defined as a transient rise in creatinine (Cr) >25% above the baseline occurs in approximately 13% of non-diabetics and in 20% of diabetics undergoing contrast procedures.[11] Fortunately, rates of CIN leading to dialysis are rare (0.5–2.0%), however, when they occur, they are related to catastrophic outcomes including a 36% in-hospital mortality rate, and a 2-year survival of only 19%.[11] Transient rises in Cr are directly related to longer intensive care unit and hospital ward stays (3 and 4 more days, respectively) after bypass surgery.[12] Recently, it has been shown that even transient rises in Cr translate to differences in adjusted long-term outcomes after PCI (Figure 2.2).[13] The leading theory is that when renal function declines, the associated abnormal vascular pathobiology accelerates, and hence the progression of CVD events occurs at a higher rate.[14]

Definition and diagnosis

Contrast-induced nephropathy usually develops within 24 to 72 hours following a radiocontrast study. This may rarely be accompanied by oliguria. One interesting feature of oliguric CIN is the presence of a low fractional excretion of sodium during the initial stages, despite no clinical evidence of volume depletion.[15]

Urinalysis shows renal tubular epithelial cell casts or coarsely granular brown casts, but may occasionally be negative. Even in the absence of a rise in serum creatinine, radiocontrast agents may still alter the urinary sediment demonstrating various degrees of abnormalities, including

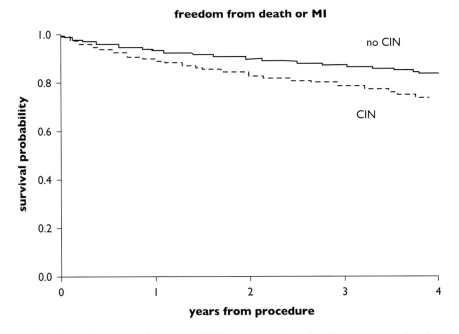

Figure 2.2 *Adjusted, long-term outcomes in 7586 patients with and without contrast-induced nephropathy (CIN) after angioplasty, P<0.0001. CIN is defined as a ≥ 0.5 mg/dl rise in creatinine after PCI. MI: myocardial infarction. (Adapted from Rihal CS et al.[13])*

the presence of epithelial cells, epithelial cell casts, granular or muddy brown coarsely granular casts, and occasional crystals.[16,17] A persistent nephrogram 24 to 48 hours after the contrast study has been reported to be a sensitive indicator of the presence of renal failure (83% of patients with renal failure had a positive nephrogram) with high specificity (93% of patients without renal failure lacked the persistent nephrogram).[18] The persistent nephrogram has been attributed to an abnormal vascular pathobiology in CKD, which causes a persistent intrarenal vasoconstriction after contrast exposure.[19–21] This vasoconstriction prolongs the dwell time of iodinated contrast in the renal parenchyma, allowing for a greater opportunity for direct cellular toxicity.

In clinical trials CIN has been variously defined as an increase in serum Cr>0.5 mg/dl (44 μmol/l)[4,13,19,22–29] or >25% of the baseline level[11,20,21,28–30] at 24,[19] 48 hours[4,13,19,22–29] or rarely >25% of the baseline level,[11,19–21,27–30] or 72,[21] 96,[30] or 120[11] hours after contrast exposure (Table 2.1). Because Cr peaks between 4 and 5 days after contrast administration,[21,31] CIN may be missed in a considerable number of patients relying on the Cr concentration assessed only up to 48 hours. Furthermore, serum Cr is an inaccurate estimate of creatinine clearance (CrCl) or estimated glomerular filtration rate (eGFR), which is better calculated according to the formula of Cockroft and Gault[32] or the modification of diet in renal disease (MDRD) study equation,[33] which is the most widely used measurement for glomerular filtration rate.

Table 2.1 Comparison of various studies involving interventions in the prevention of contrast-induced nephropathy. The incidence given is for the patients in the control group, all of whom received hydration

Author	Year	No of patients	Vascular bed	CIN definition	CIN rate (%)
Marenzi et al[34]	2003	114	Coronary and peripheral	>25% rise in sCr	50
Baker et al[30]	2003	80	Coronary	>25% rise in sCr at 48 or 72 h	21
Allaqaband et al[25]	2002	123	Coronary	Increase in sCr >0.5 mg/dl	15.3
Tumlin et al[35]	2002	51	Coronary	0.5 mg/dl or a 25% rise at 48 hours	41
Lufft et al[36]	2002	80	Renal	>25% rise or >0.5 mg/dl	7.8
Lufft et al[37]	2002	47	Renal	>25% rise at 48 h	12.8
Sabeti et al[38]	2002	85	Renal	>33% rise in 24 h	15.09
Vogt et al[31]	2001		Peripheral, renal, coronary	*HD within 1 to 6 days *>25% rise or >0.5 mg/dl	26–35
Schillinger et al[39]	2001	213	Peripheral	>20% decrease in CrCl	12.09
Erley et al[40]	1999	80	Peripheral	Increase in sCr of at least 0.5 mg/dl	3.4
Kurnik et al[41]	1998	247	Elective radiographic procedure	0.5 mg/dl or a 25% rise at 48 h	19
Lehnert et al[42]	1998	30	Peripheral and coronary	Increase of ≥0.5 mg/dl within 48 h	40%
McCullough et al[11]	1997	3695	Coronary	>25% rise	14.8
Cochran et al[43]	1983	266	Renal	>20% rise or >0.5 mg/dl	16.9

sCr: Serum creatinine; HD: hemodialysis

Cystatin C is a cationic non-glycosylated low-molecular-weight cysteine protease which is produced at a constant rate by all nucleated cells. It is not metabolized in the serum, and is freely filtered by the renal glomeruli.[44,45] Serum concentration of cystatin C has recently been reported to be superior to serum Cr with regard to assessment of GFR,[44] and to be independent of age, gender, and muscle mass.[45] In comparison with the value immediately before coronary angiography, the increase of cystatin C achieved a maximum at 24 hours after the application of the contrast agent (+7.2%). Within 48 hours, cystatin C decreased to the level before angiography. Serum Cr increased at 24 hours (+7.7%) and continued to increase at 48 hours (+11.3%). The authors concluded that serum cystatin C increases earlier after radiocontrast application compared with Cr. Therefore, cystatin C needs to be investigated as a potential early marker for nephrotoxicity, especially in the setting of short-term hospitalizations for coronary angiographies and interventions.[45] Unfortunately, there are other factors than renal function influencing cystatin C levels (e.g. malignant tumors[46] or elevation of C-reactive protein).[47] Thus, the use of cystatin C levels for measurement of GFR as well as an early marker for CIN needs to be further validated.

Acute worsening of renal function after angiography in patients with atherosclerosis may be due to cholesterol embolization rather than CIN in certain cases. The incidence of cholesterol emboli syndrome (CES) following coronary angiography has been reported to be from 0.09%[48] to 1.4%.[49] Autopsy studies report the overall prevalence of CES to be from 25% to 30% of patients following cardiac catheterization.[50] In contrast, the incidence of cholesterol embolism was 4.3% in age-matched controls who had not undergone a previous invasive vascular procedure.

In patients with CES occurring after angiographic and vascular surgical procedures, the interval from the inciting event to the onset of renal symptoms may vary greatly. Some patients have immediate clinical features, but in others the onset can be more insidious, with a delay of weeks or months between the precipitating event and clinical features. In 17 patients who developed atheroembolization after an arteriographic procedure, Scolari et al found the mean interval between the inciting event and diagnosis of atheroembolic renal disease to be 5.3 weeks.[51] Contrast-media-associated nephrotoxicity immediately follows the radiographic study. There is an increase in Cr level a few days after the procedure (usually within 72 hours); peak Cr level elevation occurs approximately 1 week after exposure and returns to baseline within 10 to 14 days.[52] Conversely, atheroembolic renal damage frequently has a delayed onset (days to weeks) and a protracted course; the outcome is often poor, resulting in progressive renal failure requiring dialysis. When a fulminant disease develops rapidly after angiography, the concomitant cutaneous, neurologic, and gastrointestinal complications usually accompany renal atheroembolic disease.[53–56]

Incidence of contrast-induced nephropathy

As is true for most other causes of acute renal failure, it has been a major challenge to compare the various studies involving radiocontrast-induced nephropathy, given the varying definitions of renal failure used in various studies. Contrast-induced nephropathy has been variously defined as either a rise in serum Cr (from baseline) of 0.3 mg/dl,[43,57] 0.5 mg/dl,[4,58,59] 0.6 mg/dl,[60] 1.0 mg/dl,[18,61–64] or 2.0 mg/dl[65,66] or a 25%[67] or 50%[68,69] increase in baseline serum Cr 1 to 5 days following exposure to radiocontrast material. D'Elia and coworkers[18] reported that 0.7% of non-azotemic patients and 17.4% of azotemic patients had a 1 mg/dl rise in serum Cr following non-renal angiography. A 12% incidence of ARF was reported in seriously ill, hospitalized patients, using a rise in serum Cr of at least 1 mg/dl within 48 hours of the study as the criterion for nephrotoxicity[70] (see Table 2.1). Considering numerous definitions in numerous studies, the incidence of CIN in the general population undergoing radiographic procedures with iodinated contrast is approximately 15%.

Risk factors for contrast-induced nephropathy

Mild, transient decreases in GFR occur after contrast administration in almost all patients.[71] Whether a patient develops clinically significant acute renal failure, however, depends very much on the presence or absence of certain risk factors (Table 2.2). A multivariate analysis of prospective trials has shown that baseline renal impairment, diabetes mellitus, congestive heart failure, and higher doses of contrast media increase the risk of CIN.[72] Other risk factors include reduced effective arterial volume (e.g. due to dehydration, nephrosis, cirrhosis) or concurrent use of potentially nephrotoxic drugs such as non-steroidal anti-inflammatory agents and angiotensin-converting enzyme inhibitors. Multiple myeloma has been suggested as a potential risk factor for CIN, but a large retrospective study failed to demonstrate an increased risk in these patients.[73] Of all these risk factors, pre-existing renal impairment appears to be the single most important; patients with diabetes mellitus and renal impairment, however, have a substantially higher risk of CIN than patients with renal impairment alone.[69,74]

A direct toxic effect of contrast media on renal epithelial cells has been shown,[75] as well as an increased red cell aggregation, possibly further impairing oxygen delivery.[76] Experimental studies on the role of osmolality *per se* in the pathogenesis of CIN have provided conflicting data.[76–78] Clinical trials indicate a lower incidence of CIN when using low-osmolality compared with high-osmolality contrast agents,[74,79] and when using iodixanol compared to a low-osmolal agents, iohexol.[80] A large study comparing the low-osmolality agent iohexol to the high-osmolality agent diatrizoate in patients with pre-existing renal dysfunction undergoing angiography found a lower incidence of CIN (defined as an increase in serum Cr > 0.5 mg/dl within 48 to 72 hours) in the iohexol group (12.2%) than in the diatrizoate group (27%). This effect was even more evident in patients with both renal dysfunction and diabetes.[74] The incidence of CIN (defined as an increase in serum Cr > 0.5 mg/dl within 3 days) in patients with both diabetes and pre-existing renal dysfunction was recently reported to be markedly lower when using the iso-osmolar, non-ionic contrast agent iodixanol (3%) compared with iohexol (26%).[80] Nevertheless, additional and possibly larger studies are needed to understand whether the use of iso-osmolar agents may be of benefit compared to other low-osmolar contrast agents.

Table 2.2 Risk factors for the development of contrast-induced nephropathy	
• eGFR ≤ 60 ml/min per 1.73 m²	• Congestive heart failure
• Diabetes	• Periprocedural volume depletion
• Urine ACR > 30	• Intraprocedural hypotension
• Hypertension	• Intra-aortic counterpulsation
• History of structural kidney disease or damage	• Cholesterol emboli syndrome
	• Use of large volume of contrast
ACR: urine albumin–creatinine ratio; eGFR: estimated glomerular filtration rate.	

Prediction of contrast-induced nephropathy

Chronic kidney disease is defined through a range of eGFR values by the National Kidney Foundation Kidney Disease Outcomes Quality Initiative (KDOQI) as depicted in Figure 2.3.[7] Most studies of cardiovascular outcomes have found that a breakpoint for the development of CIN, later restenosis, recurrent myocardial infarction (MI), diastolic/systolic congestive heart failure (CHF), and cardiovascular death occurs below an eGFR of 60 ml/min per 1.73 m^2, which roughly corresponds to a serum Cr of > 1.5 mg/dl in the general population.[81–84] Because Cr is a crude indicator of renal function, and often underestimates renal dysfunction in women and the elderly, calculated measures of eGFR or CrCl by the Cockroft–Gault equation or by the MDRD equations, now available on the web, personal digital assistants, and with hand-held plastic estimators are the preferred methods of estimating renal function. The four-variable MDRD equation for estimated GFR is the preferred method since it does not rely on body weight.[85] This equation is given below:

$$\text{GFR} = (186.3 \times [\text{serum creatinine}^{-1.154}] \times [\text{age}^{-0.203}])$$

calculated values are multiplied by 0.742 for women and by 1.21 for African Americans. In addition, microalbuminuria (defined as a random urine albumin/creatinine ratio (ACR) of 30–300 mg/g) at any level of eGFR is considered to represent CKD, and has been thought

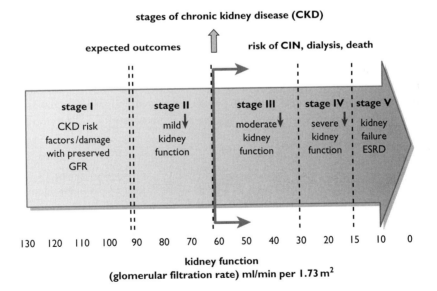

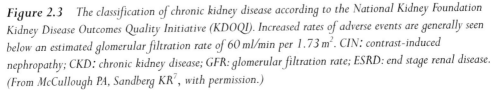

Figure 2.3 *The classification of chronic kidney disease according to the National Kidney Foundation Kidney Disease Outcomes Quality Initiative (KDOQI). Increased rates of adverse events are generally seen below an estimated glomerular filtration rate of 60 ml/min per 1.73 m^2. CIN: contrast-induced nephropathy; CKD: chronic kidney disease; GFR: glomerular filtration rate; ESRD: end stage renal disease. (From McCullough PA, Sandberg KR[7], with permission.)*

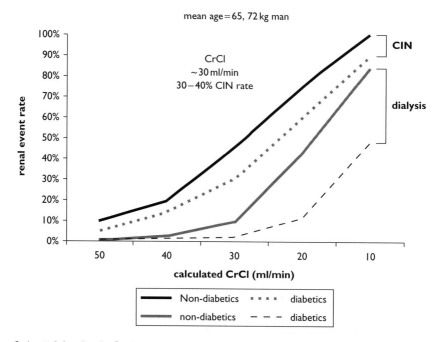

mean age = 65, 72 kg man

CrCl
~30 ml/min
30–40% CIN rate

renal event rate

calculated CrCl (ml/min)

CIN

dialysis

| Non-diabetics | · · · · diabetics |
| non-diabetics | – – – diabetics |

Figure 2.4 *Validated risk of radiocontrast nephropathy and dialysis after diagnostic angiography and ad-hoc angioplasty by creatinine clearance (CrCl) and diabetes. This assumes a mean contrast dose of 250 ml and a mean age of 65. (From McCullough PA, Sandberg KR[7], with permission.)*

to occur as the result of endothelial dysfunction in the glomeruli.[86] It is critical to understand that the risk of CIN is related in a curvilinear fashion to the eGFR, as shown in Figure 2.4.[8] Multivariate prediction scoring schemes have been developed and indicate that patients with multiple risk factors can have a very high, if not certain expectation for the development of CIN after contrast exposure during PCI (Figure 2.5).[88] This validated scoring scheme can be used to anticipate CIN before and immediately after coronary angiography. As Figure 2.5 implies, elderly, diabetic patients with reduced eGFR or elevated Cr, with additional risk features, can have CIN and ARF requiring dialysis rates as high as 57 and 16%, respectively. Hence, this type of scheme can be used in the informed consent process, prevention planning, and anticipation of the need for dialysis after the procedure.

The most important risk factor for CIN is pre-existing renal dysfunction.[8,11,13] The presence of diabetes mellitus has significant impact on the incidence of CIN in patients with mild-to-moderate renal insufficiency (Cr < 2.0 mg/dl), whereas, in patients with advanced renal insufficiency (Cr ≥ 2.0 mg/dl), the incidence of CIN in patients with diabetic and non-diabetic nephropathy does not differ.[13] The degree of pre-existing renal impairment is the most powerful predictor of CIN, and patients with atherosclerosis and reduced effective circulating arterial volume are at particular risk (Table 2.3). Peripheral vascular disease, bypass graft intervention, and the need for an intra-aortic

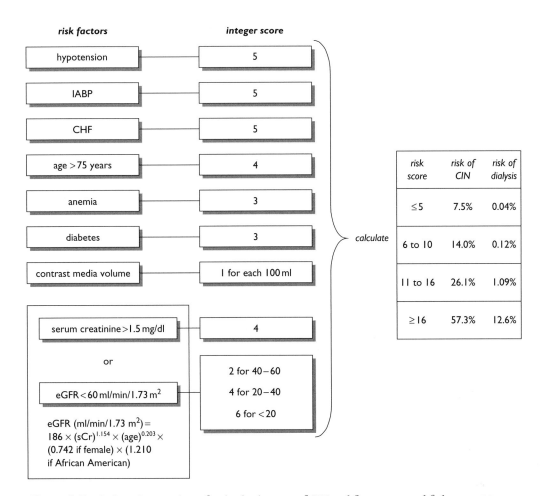

Figure 2.5 *Risk prediction scheme for the development of CIN and for serious renal failure requiring dialysis. Anemia: baseline hematocrit value < 39% for men and < 36% for women; CHF: congestive heart failure functional class III/IV, and/or history of pulmonary edema; eGFR: estimated glomerular filtration rate; hypotension: systolic blood pressure < 80 mm Hg for at least 1 hour requiring inotropic support with medications or intra-aortic balloon pump (IABP) within 24 h peri-procedurally. (From Mehran R, Aymong ED, Nikolsky E et al[88], with permission.)*

balloon pump probably are surrogates of more severe atherosclerosis and advanced and long-lasting coronary artery disease. Procedures with bypass graft angiography and intervention may be associated with higher complexity, longer duration, and limited success, thus indicating an unstable post-procedural period with impaired cardiac output. In addition, older age, hypertension, repeated exposure to contrast medium, and nephrotoxic medication, such as aminoglycosides, as well as drugs impairing the renovascular autoregulation such as NSAIDs and angiotensin-converting enzyme inhibitors were reported to be risk factors.[89]

27

Table 2.3 Independent predictors for the development of contrast nephropathy

Risk factor	Odds ratio	95% Confidence interval	Reference*
Contrast nephropathy†			
Pre-existing renal failure			
Preprocedural creatinine 2.0–2.9 mg/dl	7.37	4.78–11.39	13
Preprocedural creatinine ≥3 mg/dl	12.82	8.01–20.54	13
Diabetes	1.61	1.21–2.16	13
Creatinine 0–1.1 mg/dl	1.86	1.20–2.89	13
Creatinine 1.2–1.9 mg/dl	2.42	1.54–3.79	13
Creatinine 2.0–2.9 mg/dl	1.00	0.48–2.08	13
Creatinine ≥3.0	1.36	0.63–2.92	13
Preprocedure shock	1.19	0.72–1.96	13
Myocardial infarction ≤24 h	1.85	1.31–2.63	13
Congestive heart failure	1.53	1.21–2.10	13
Peripheral vascular disease	1.71	1.23–2.37	13
Contrast volume			
Total contrast volume (per 100 ml)	1.12	1.02–1.23	13
Contrast nephropathy requiring dialysis			
Chronic renal insufficiency§	20.25	11.48–35.71	8
Diabetes	3.34	1.92–5.81	8
	5.47	1.40–21.32	11
Contrast volume	1.10	1.0003–1.22	8
	1.008	1.002–1.013	11
Intra-aortic balloon pump	1.94	1.08–3.49	8
Bypass graft intervention	4.94	1.16–20.9	8

*Data are mainly derived from two studies[8,13] restricted to patients undergoing percutaneous coronary interventions and not only diagnostic angiography.
†Defined as increase in serum creatinine >0.5 mg/dl from preprocedural values.
§Defined as the presence of previously documented renal insufficiency or a baseline creatinine level of at least 1.8 mg/dl (159.1 μmol/l).
Table modified from Maeder M et al.[91]

Contrast-induced nephropathy is rare in patients with normal renal function in the absence of diabetes mellitus.[13,74] Rihal et al[13] found a 2% incidence of CIN in non-diabetic patients with a baseline $Cr \le 1.1$ mg/dl. On the other hand, 50% of patients with diabetic nephropathy and a mean serum Cr of 5.9 mg/dl had a > 25% increase after coronary angiography.[90] Hence, the degree of risk and the incidence of CIN always depend on the population studied. The use of multivariate risk prediction schemes has improved our ability to predict and, hopefully, with good management prevent some cases of CIN. Newer and better markers of eGFR including cystatin C may be able to fine-tune our approach to risk prediction in the future.

Conclusion

Contrast-induced nephropathy is an important cause of ARF and death in patients undergoing procedures with iodinated contrast. The presence of multiple risk factors can anticipate an approximate 50% probability of CIN in any given patient. Risk prediction and preventive measures are mandatory. Once ARF occurs, dialysis and expectant management are associated with high rates of in-hospital and long-term mortality.

References

1. Cotton DB. Radiocontrast-induced renal failure. *Lancet* 1979; **2**:1378–9.
2. Radiocontrast-induced renal failure. *Lancet* 1979; **2**:835. (No authors listed)
3. Heyman SN, Rosen S, Brezis M. Radiocontrast nephropathy: a paradigm for the synergism between toxic and hypoxic insults in the kidney. *Exp Nephrol* 1994; **2**:153–7.
4. Solomon R, Werner C, Mann D et al. Effects of saline, mannitol, and furosemide to prevent acute decreases in renal function induced by radiocontrast agents. *N Engl J Med* 1994; **331**:1416–20.
5. Nash K, Hafeez A, Hou S. Hospital-acquired renal insufficiency. *Am J Kidney Dis* 2002; **39**:930–6.
6. Taylor AJ, Hotchkiss D, Morse D et al. PREPARED: Preparation for Angiography in Renal Dysfunction: a randomized trial of inpatient vs outpatient hydration protocols for cardiac catheterization in mild-to-moderate renal dysfunction. *Chest* 1998; **114**:1570–4.
7. McCullough PA, Sandberg KR. Epidemiology of contrast-induced nephropathy. *Rev Cardiovasc Med* 2003; **4(Suppl 5)**:S3–9.
8. Gruberg L, Mehran R, Dangas G. Acute renal failure requiring dialysis after percutaneous coronary interventions. *Catheter Cardiovasc Interv* 2001; **52**:409–16.
9. Lewis CE, Jacobs DR Jr, McCreath H et al. Weight gain continues in the 1990s: 10-year trends in weight and overweight from the CARDIA study. Coronary Artery Risk Development in Young Adults. *Am J Epidemiol* 2000; **151**:1172–81.
10. Bakris GL, Williams M, Dworkin L et al. Preserving renal function in adults with hypertension and diabetes: a consensus approach. National Kidney Foundation Hypertension and Diabetes Executive Committees Working Group. *Am J Kidney Dis* 2000; **36**:646–61.
11. McCullough PA, Wolyn R, Rocher LL et al. Acute renal failure after coronary intervention: incidence, risk factors, and relationship to mortality. *Am J Med* 1997; **103**:368–75.
12. Mangano CM, Diamondstone LS, Ramsay JG et al. Renal dysfunction after myocardial revascularization: risk factors, adverse outcomes, and hospital resource utilization. The Multicenter Study of Perioperative Ischemia Research Group. *Ann Intern Med* 1998; **128**:194–203.

13. Rihal CS, Textor SC, Grill DE et al. Incidence and prognostic importance of acute renal failure after percutaneous coronary intervention. *Circulation* 2002; **105**:2259–64.

14. McCullough PA. Cardiorenal risk: an important clinical intersection. *Rev Cardiovasc Med* 2002; **3**:71–6.

15. Fang LS, Sirota RA, Ebert TH et al. Low fractional excretion of sodium with contrast media-induced acute renal failure. *Arch Intern Med* 1980; **140**:531–3.

16. Gelman ML, Coggins CH et al. Effects of an angiographic contrast agent on renal function. *Cardiovasc Med* 1979; **4**:313.

17. Weinrauch LA, Healy RW, Leland OS Jr et al. Coronary angiography and acute renal failure in diabetic azotemic nephropathy. *Ann Intern Med* 1977; **86**:56–9.

18. D'Elia JA, Gleason RE, Alday M et al. Nephrotoxicity from angiographic contrast material. A prospective study. *Am J Med* 1982; **72**:719–25.

19. Diaz-Sandoval LJ, Kosowsky BD, Losordo DW. Acetylcysteine to prevent angiography-related renal tissue injury (the APART trial). *Am J Cardiol* 2002; **89**:356–8.

20. Kay J, Chow WH, Chan TM et al. Acetylcysteine for prevention of acute deterioration of renal function following elective coronary angiography and intervention: a randomized controlled trial. *JAMA* 2003; **289**:553–8.

21. MacNeill BD, Harding SA, Bazari H et al. Prophylaxis of contrast-induced nephropathy in patients undergoing coronary angiography. *Catheter Cardiovasc Interven* 2003; **60**:458–61.

22. Mueller C, Buerkle G, Buettner HJ et al. Prevention of contrast media-associated nephropathy: randomized comparison of 2 hydration regimens in 1620 patients undergoing coronary angioplasty. *Arch Intern Med* 2002; **162**:329–36.

23. Durham JD, Caputo C, Dokko J et al. A randomized controlled trial of N-acetylcysteine to prevent contrast nephropathy in cardiac angiography. *Kidney Int* 2002; **62**:2202–7.

24. Boccalandro F, Amhad M, Smalling RW et al. Oral acetylcysteine does not protect renal function from moderate to high doses of intravenous radiographic contrast. *Catheter Cardiovasc Interven* 2003; **58**:336–41.

25. Allaqaband S, Tumuluri R, Malik AM et al. Prospective randomized study of N-acetylcysteine, fenoldopam, and saline for prevention of radiocontrast-induced nephropathy. *Catheter Cardiovasc Interven* 2002; **57**:279–83.

26. Goldenberg I, Shechter M, Matetzky S et al. Oral acetylcysteine as an adjunct to saline hydration for the prevention of contrast-induced nephropathy following coronary angiography. A randomized controlled trial and review of the current literature. *Eur Heart J* 2004; **25**:212–18.

27. Shyu KG, Cheng JJ, Kuan P. Acetylcysteine protects against acute renal damage in patients with abnormal renal function undergoing a coronary procedure. *J Am Coll Cardiol* 2002; **40**:1383–8.

28. Briguori C, Colombo A, Violante A et al. Standard vs double dose of N-acetylcysteine to prevent contrast agent associated nephrotoxicity. *Eur Heart J* 2004; **25**:206–11.

29. Oldemeyer JB, Biddle WP, Wurdeman RL et al. Acetylcysteine in the prevention of contrast-induced nephropathy after coronary angiography. *Am Heart J* 2003; **146**:E23.

30. Baker CS, Wragg A, Kumar S et al. A rapid protocol for the prevention of contrast-induced renal dysfunction: the RAPPID study. *J Am Coll Cardiol*, 2003; **41**:2114–18.

31. Vogt B, Ferrari P, Schonholzer C et al. Prophylactic hemodialysis after radiocontrast media in patients with renal insufficiency is potentially harmful. *Am J Med* 2001; **111**:692–8.

32. Cockcroft DW, Gault MH. Prediction of creatinine clearance from serum creatinine. *Nephron* 1976; **16**:31–41.

33. Levey AS, Bosch JP, Lewis JB et al. A more accurate method to estimate glomerular filtration rate from serum creatinine: a new prediction equation. Modification of Diet in Renal Disease Study Group. *Ann Intern Med* 1999; **130**:461–70.

34. Marenzi G, Marana I, Lauri G et al. The prevention of radiocontrast-agent-induced nephropathy by hemofiltration. *N Engl J Med* 2003; **349**:1331–8.

35. Tumlin JA et al. Fenoldopam mesylate blocks reductions in renal plasma flow after radiocontrast dye infusion: a pilot trial in the prevention of contrast nephropathy. *Am Heart J* 2002; **143**: 894–903.

36. Lufft V, Hoogestraat-Lufft L, Fels LM et al. Contrast media nephropathy: intravenous CT angiography versus intraarterial digital subtraction angiography in renal artery stenosis: a prospective randomized trial. *Am J Kidney Dis* 2002; **40**:236–42.

37. Lufft V, Hoogestraat-Lufft L, Fels LM et al. Angiography for renal artery stenosis: no additional impairment of renal function by angioplasty. *Eur Radiol* 2002; **12**:804–9.

38. Sabeti S, Schillinger M, Mlekusch W et al. Reduction in renal function after renal arteriography and after renal artery angioplasty. *Eur J Vasc Endovasc Surg* 2002; **24**:156–60.

39. Schillinger M, Haumer M, Mlekusch W et al. Predicting renal failure after balloon angioplasty in high-risk patients. *J Endovasc Ther* 2001; **8**:609–14.

40. Erley CM, Duda SH, Rehfuss D et al. Prevention of radiocontrast-media-induced nephropathy in patients with pre-existing renal insufficiency by hydration in combination with the adenosine antagonist theophylline. *Nephrol Dial Transplant* 1999; **14**:1146–9.

41. Kurnik BR, Allgren RL, Genter FC et al. Prospective study of atrial natriuretic peptide for the prevention of radiocontrast-induced nephropathy. *Am J Kidney Dis* 1998; **31**: 674–80.

42. Lehnert T, Keller E, Gondolf K et al. Effect of haemodialysis after contrast medium administration in patients with renal insufficiency. *Nephrol Dial Transplant* 1998; **13**:358–62.

43. Cochran ST, Wong WS, Roe DJ. Predicting angiography-induced acute renal function impairment: clinical risk model. *AJR* 1983; **141**:1027–33.

44. Dharnidharka VR, Kwon C, Stevens G. Serum cystatin C is superior to serum creatinine as a marker of kidney function: a meta-analysis. *Am J Kidney Dis* 2002; **40**:221–6.

45. Rickli H, Benou K, Ammann P et al. Time course of serial cystatin C levels in comparison with serum creatinine after application of radiocontrast media. *Clin Nephrol* 2004; **61**:98–102.

46. Page MK, Bukki J, Luppa P et al. Clinical value of cystatin C determination. *Clin Chim Acta* 2000; **297**:67–72.

47. Knight EL, Verhave JC, Spiegelman D et al. Factors influencing serum cystatin C levels other than renal function and the impact on renal function measurement. *Kidney Int* 2004; **65**:1416–21.

48. Scolari F, Bracchi M, Valzorio B et al. Cholesterol atheromatous embolism: an increasingly recognized cause of acute renal failure. *Nephrol Dial Transplant* 1996; **11**:1607–12.

49. Fukumoto Y, Tsutsui H, Tsuchihashi M et al. The incidence and risk factors of cholesterol embolization syndrome, a complication of cardiac catheterization: a prospective study. *J Am Coll Cardiol* 2003; **42**:211–16.

50. Rosansky SJ, Deschamps EG. Multiple cholesterol emboli syndrome after angiography. *Am J Med Sci* 1984; **288**:45–8.

51. Scolari F, Tardanico R, Zani R et al. Cholesterol crystal embolism: a recognizable cause of renal disease. *Am J Kidney Dis* 2000; **36**:1089–109.

52. Rudnick MR, Berns JS, Cohen RM et al. Nephrotoxic risks of renal angiography: contrast media-associated nephrotoxicity and atheroembolism – a critical review. *Am J Kidney Dis* 1994; **24**:713–27.

53. Kassirer JP. Atheroembolic renal disease. *N Engl J Med* 1969; **280**:812–18.

54. Fine MJ, Kapoor W, Falanga V. Cholesterol crystal embolization: a review of 221 cases in the English literature. *Angiology* 1987; **38**:769–84.

55. Saleem S, Lakkis FG, Martinez-Maldonado M. Atheroembolic renal disease. *Semin Nephrol* 1996; **16**:309–18.

56. Dahlberg PJ, Frecentese DF, Cogbill TH. Cholesterol embolism: experience with 22 histologically proven cases. *Surgery* 1989; **105**:737–46.

57. Older RA, Korobkin M, Cleeve DM et al. Contrast-induced acute renal failure: persistent nephrogram as clue to early detection. *AJR* 1980; **134**:339–42.

58. Powe NR, Steinberg EP, Erikson JE et al. Contrast medium-induced adverse reactions: economic outcome. *Radiology* 1988; **169**:163–8.

59. Schwab SJ, Hlatky MA, Pieper KS et al. Contrast nephrotoxicity: a randomized controlled trial of a nonionic and an ionic radiographic contrast agent. *N Engl J Med* 1989; **320**:149–53.

60. Older RA, Miller JP, Jackson DC et al. Angiographically induced renal failure and its radiographic detection. *AJR* 1976; **126**:1039–45.

61. Cigarroa RG, Lange RA, Hillis LD et al. Dosing of contrast material to prevent contrast nephropathy in patients with renal disease. *Am J Med* 1989; **86(6 pt 1)**:649–52.

62. Eisenberg RL, Bank WO, Hedgcock MW. Renal failure after major angiography. *Am J Med* 1980; **68**:43–6.

63. Harkonen S, Kjellstrand CM. Exacerbation of diabetic renal failure following intravenous pyelography. *Am J Med* 1977; **63**:939–46.

64. Levitz CS, Friedman EA. Failure of protective measures to prevent contrast media-induced renal failure. *Arch Intern Med* 1982; **142**:642–3.

65. Byrd L, Sherman RL. Radiocontrast-induced acute renal failure: a clinical and pathophysiologic review. *Medicine (Baltimore)* 1979; **58**:270–9.

66. Carvallo A, Rakowski TA, Argy WP et al. Acute renal failure following drip infusion pyelography. *Am J Med* 1978; **65**:38–45.

67. Weisberg LS, Kurnik PB, Kurnik BR. Risk of radiocontrast nephropathy in patients with and without diabetes mellitus. *Kidney Int* 1994; **45**:259–65.

68. Cramer BC, Parfrey PS, Hutchinson TA et al. Renal function following infusion of radiologic contrast material. A prospective controlled study. *Arch Intern Med* 1985; **145**:87–9.

69. Parfrey PS, Griffiths SM, Barrett BJ et al. Contrast material-induced renal failure in patients with diabetes mellitus, renal insufficiency, or both. A prospective controlled study. *N Engl J Med* 1989; **320**:143–9.

70. Swartz RD, Rubin JE, Leeming BW et al. Renal failure following major angiography. *Am J Med* 1978; **65**:31–7.

71. Katholi RE, Taylor GJ, McCann WP et al. Nephrotoxicity from contrast media: attenuation with theophylline. *Radiology* 1995; **195**:17–22.

72. Barrett BJ. Contrast nephrotoxicity. *J Am Soc Nephrol* 1994; **5**:125–37.

73. McCarthy CS, Becker JA. Multiple myeloma and contrast media. *Radiology* 1992; **183**:519–21.

74. Rudnick MR, Goldfarb S, Wexler L et al. Nephrotoxicity of ionic and nonionic contrast media in 1196 patients: a randomized trial. The Iohexol Cooperative Study. *Kidney Int* 1995; **47**:254–61.

75. Humes HD, Hunt DA, White MD. Direct toxic effect of the radiocontrast agent diatrizoate on renal proximal tubule cells. *Am J Physiol* 1987; **252(2 Pt 2)**:F246–55.

76. Liss P, Nygren A, Olsson U et al. Effects of contrast media and mannitol on renal medullary blood flow and red cell aggregation in the rat kidney. *Kidney Int* 1996; **49**:1268–75.

77. Hizoh I, Strater J, Schick CS et al. Radiocontrast-induced DNA fragmentation of renal tubular cells in vitro: role of hypertonicity. *Nephrol Dial Transplant* 1998; **13**:911–18.

78. Deray G, Bagnis C, Jacquiaud C et al. Renal effects of low and isoosmolar contrast media on renal hemodynamic in a normal and ischemic dog kidney. *Invest Radiol* 1999; **34**:1–4.

79. Barrett BJ, Carlisle EJ. Metaanalysis of the relative nephrotoxicity of high- and low-osmolality iodinated contrast media. *Radiology* 1993; **188**:171–8.

80. Aspelin P, Aubry P, Fransson SG et al. Nephrotoxic effects in high-risk patients undergoing angiography. *N Engl J Med* 2003; **348**:491–9.
81. McCullough PA, Soman SS, Shah SS et al. Risks associated with renal dysfunction in patients in the coronary care unit. *J Am Coll Cardiol* 2000; **36**:679–84.
82. Beattie JN, Soman SS, Sandberg KR et al. Determinants of mortality after myocardial infarction in patients with advanced renal dysfunction. *Am J Kidney Dis* 2001; **37**:1191–200.
83. Chertow GM, Lazarus JM, Christiansen CL et al. Preoperative renal risk stratification. *Circulation* 1997; **95**:878–84.
84. Szczech LA, Best PJ, Crowley E et al. Outcomes of patients with chronic renal insufficiency in the bypass angioplasty revascularization investigation. *Circulation* 2002; **105**:2253–8.
85. National Kidney Foundation. K/DOQI clinical practice guidelines for chronic kidney disease: evaluation, classification, and stratification. *Am J Kidney Dis* 2002; **39(2 Suppl 1)**:S1–266.
86. Keane WF, Eknoyan G. Proteinuria, albuminuria, risk, assessment, detection, elimination (PARADE): a position paper of the National Kidney Foundation. *Am J Kidney Dis* 1999; **33**:1004–10.
87. McCullough PA, Manley HJ. Prediction and prevention of contrast nephropathy. *J Interven Cardiol* 2001; **14**:547–58.
88. Mehran R, Aymong ED, Nikolsky E et al. A simple risk score for prediction of contrast-induced nephropathy after percutaneous coronary intervention: development and initial validation. *J Am Coll Cardiol* 2004; **44**:1393–9.
89. Huber W, Schipek C, Ilgmann K et al. Effectiveness of theophylline prophylaxis of renal impairment after coronary angiography in patients with chronic renal insufficiency. *Am J Cardiol* 2003; **91**:1157–62.
90. Manske CL, Sprafka JM, Strony JT et al. Contrast nephropathy in azotemic diabetic patients undergoing coronary angiography. *Am J Med* 1990; **89**:615–20.
91. Maeder M, Klein M, Rickli H et al. Contrast nephropathy: review focusing on prevention. *J Am Coll Cardiol* 2004; **44**:1763–71.

3. CLINICAL FEATURES AND PROGNOSTIC IMPLICATIONS OF CONTRAST-INDUCED NEPHROPATHY

Luis Gruberg

Introduction

The significant advances that have occurred in the field of interventional cardiology in the last decade with the introduction and popularization of stents and platelet inhibitors have led to an exponential increase in the number of catheter-based procedures currently performed around the world. Despite the undisputable benefit that these techniques offer to patients, there are still limitations. It is important to remember that the use of radiocontrast material during percutaneous coronary intervention (PCI) is associated with a risk of developing acute contrast-induced nephropathy (CIN), the third leading cause of hospital-acquired renal insufficiency. Despite the fact that numerous preventative methods have been explored to prevent CIN, it continues to be a source of concern, particularly in patients with pre-existing renal insufficiency who need to undergo contrast-enhanced radiographic examinations and interventions. In patients with normal renal function, CIN is relatively rare, but its frequency increases in patients with abnormal renal function with or without diabetes mellitus, and all the more in patients with a combination of both diseases. Unfortunately, patients who develop CIN during PCI face a poor prognosis; the condition is associated with high rates of morbidity, mortality, resource utilization, and prolonged hospitalization.

Definition

Many definitions of CIN are available in the literature, but the two most common include a rise in serum creatinine $\geq 25\%$ from baseline or an absolute increase of > 0.5 mg/dl from baseline. In the majority of patients, this rise occurs within the first 24 hours, peaking 3–4 days after the procedure, and is coupled with a reduction in creatinine clearance (CrCl).[1] Various institutions have adopted this definition of CIN as a threshold to determine whether the discharge of a patient should be delayed.[2] Unfortunately, serum creatinine measurement is an insensitive method to monitor renal function, as $> 50\%$ reduction in glomerular filtration rate (GFR) may occur before any increase is observed. Furthermore, the nadir of renal dysfunction occurs 3 to 5 days after contrast exposure and, in most cases, returns to normal within 7 to 10 days. A more accurate way to assess the renal function may be to calculate the CrCl by applying the Cockcroft–Gault equation or by calculating the GFR using the Modification of Diet in Renal Disease (MDRD) formula.[3]

Recently published guidelines have redefined chronic kidney disease, an important risk factor for cardiovascular disease, especially in endstage renal disease patients on dialysis replacement therapy.[4] These patients have mortality rates that are 10 to 30 times higher than in the general population and are now considered to be in the highest risk group for subsequent cardiovascular events.[4,5]

Clinical characteristics

It is important to note that patients who undergo PCI nowadays are usually discharged within <24 hours of the procedure, and they may develop this complication at home. Although the clinical importance of CIN may not be immediately obvious given the subclinical course and the high frequency of recovery of renal function, it is by no means a benign complication. CIN is no different from acute renal failure of any other etiology in terms of the symptoms, signs, complications that may ensue, and prognostic implications. It is the third most common cause of acute tubular necrosis in patients admitted to hospital. Some degree of residual renal impairment has been reported in as many as 30% of those affected and up to 7% may require temporary dialysis or progress to endstage renal failure.[6–8] Proteinuria and oliguria may be observed in some patients, especially in those with prior renal insufficiency. However, CIN is usually non-oliguric and reversible. The serum creatinine level usually increases within 24–48 hours after contrast media administration, reaches a peak value at 3–5 days (generally an increase of 0.5–3.0 mg/dl), and then returns to baseline within 7–10 days.[9,10] Urinalysis is often compatible with acute tubular necrosis, demonstrating renal tubular epithelial cells and coarse granular casts.[7] In high-risk patients, CIN may present as a more severe acute renal failure. In these patients, oliguria may develop within 24 hours of contrast administration, with peak levels of serum creatinine exceeding 5 mg/dl, sometimes requiring dialysis. As discussed previously, permanent renal damage that requires dialysis replacement therapy is an unusual complication, but with dire consequences.[1,11,12] In a study from the Washington Hospital Center, 0.7% of patients who underwent PCI required dialysis. These patients were usually older, female, diabetics, and 61% had prior history of chronic kidney disease.[11] At 1-year follow-up, only 45% were alive and 75% of them required permanent dialysis replacement therapy. Similar results were described by McCullough et al, in which the in-hospital mortality of these patients was 35.7%.[1] It is important to note that the majority of these patients suffer from generalized atherosclerotic vascular disease and may be at an increased risk to develop acute renal failure secondary to atheroembolic disease.[12] Acute renal failure secondary to atheroembolic disease usually presents later, approximately 7 days to weeks; it is usually associated with a brief period of eosinophilia, hypocomplementemia, and other evidence of embolic phenomena, including livedo reticularis and/or gastrointestinal ischemia or infarction. The course of this disease is more prolonged and usually there is no recovery of renal function.

Prognostic implications

The occurrence of CIN may prolong in-hospital stay and is associated with an increase in morbidity, mortality, and costs. The prognosis is especially unfavorable in patients with prior renal disease.[13–16] In a study of 1826 consecutive patients who underwent coronary intervention at the William Beaumont Hospital, McCullough and colleagues showed that CIN occurred in 14.5% of these patients and only 0.8% of all patients developed CIN that required dialysis.[1] In-hospital mortality was 7.1% and 35.7%, respectively (Figure 3.1). As we can observe, only a small minority of patients had deterioration in renal function that required dialysis; nevertheless, at 2-year follow-up, the mortality rate for these patients was 81.2% (Figure 3.2).

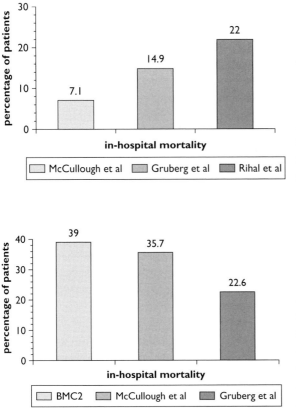

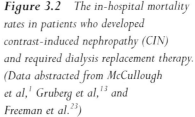

Figure 3.1 The in-hospital mortality rates in patients who developed contrast-induced nephropathy. (From McCullough et al,[1] Gruberg et al,[13] and Rihal et al.[21])

Figure 3.2 The in-hospital mortality rates in patients who developed contrast-induced nephropathy (CIN) and required dialysis replacement therapy. (Data abstracted from McCullough et al,[1] Gruberg et al,[13] and Freeman et al.[23])

A study from the Washington Hospital Center in 439 consecutive patients revealed that the incidence of CIN (defined as an increase in serum creatinine $\geq 25\%$ within 48 hours) was 37%.[13] It is important to note that these patients had chronic kidney disease (not on dialysis replacement therapy) with a baseline serum creatinine level ≥ 1.8 mg/dl. In-hospital mortality rate was 14.9% for patients who developed CIN, compared to only 4.9% in patients who did not develop this complication (Figures 4.1 and 4.3). Furthermore, in-hospital mortality for patients who required dialysis (7% of the whole cohort) was 22.6% and, among them, four patients required permanent dialysis replacement therapy (Figure 3.2). The in-hospital course of patients who developed CIN was characterized by increased morbidity, with a significantly higher rate of myocardial infarction, pulmonary edema, gastro-intestinal bleeding, and need for subsequent blood transfusion (Figure 3.3). The cumulative 1-year mortality was 37.7% for patients with CIN and 45.2% for those who developed CIN and required dialysis (Figures 4.2 and 4.4).[13]

Another study from the same group assessed the long-term outcomes of 5967 patients with no history of renal insufficiency and a baseline serum creatinine of ≤ 1.2 mg/dl who underwent PCI between 1994 and 2000.[16] In this study, Lindsay and colleagues showed that 208 patients (3.5%) developed CIN (defined as an increase in serum creatinine $\geq 50\%$ of the baseline value). Renal dysfunction was severe enough to require dialysis in only three patients. As usual, patients who

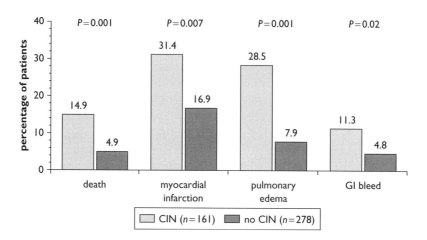

Figure 3.3 *The in-hospital outcomes of patients who developed contrast-induced nephropathy (CIN) (□) and those who did not (■). (Data abstracted from Gruberg et al.[13])*

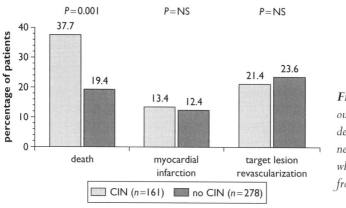

Figure 3.4 *The 1-year outcomes of patients who developed contrast-induced nephropathy (CIN) (□) and those who did not (■). (Data abstracted from Gruberg et al.[13])*

developed CIN were older, more often female, hypertensive, and had a higher incidence of diabetes mellitus and peripheral vascular disease. These patients received a higher volume of contrast material and a greater number of stenoses were treated at the same time. The in-hospital course of these patients was marked by a significant increase in pulmonary edema, neurologic events, bleeding, and vascular complications. For the purpose of the long-term analysis, the investigators excluded from the study all patients with a major in-hospital complication such as death, myocardial infarction, or urgent coronary artery bypass surgery. At 1-year follow-up, the cumulative mortality was more than three times as frequent, and postdischarge myocardial infarction more than twice, as was the incidence of target vessel revascularization in those patients with CIN (Figure 3.5). Gupta and colleagues observed similar results in a registry of 9067 patients who underwent PCI at the Cleveland Clinic.[17] In this study, 143 patients developed CIN (defined as an

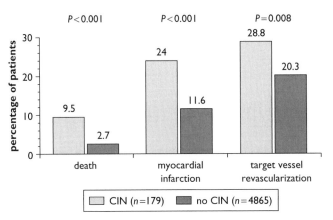

Figure 3.5 The 1-year outcomes of patients who developed contrast-induced nephropathy (CIN) (□) and those who did not (■) in the study by Lindsay et al.[16]

increase in serum creatinine >1 mg/dl) after the procedure. The 1- and 2-year mortality rate for these patients was 29.7% and 35.8% compared to 6.4% and 9.3% for patients who did not develop CIN (*P*<0.0001). Even among patients with a baseline creatinine of <1.5 mg/dl, mortality rates were higher in those patients who developed CIN compared to those with no CIN. Conversely, in patients with serum creatinine levels >1.5 mg/dl the mortality rate was 27% among those without CIN and 63.5% in patients developing this complication after PCI.

Previous studies have shown that an increase in serum creatine phosphokinase-MB (CK-MB) following PCI is associated with a higher risk of death, myocardial infarction, and revascularization procedures, even in the absence of clinically recognized abrupt vessel closure.[18,19] High-risk patients with complex target lesions, extensive atherosclerotic plaque burden, saphenous vein graft disease, advanced age, or multivessel disease have all been linked to elevated CK-MB levels after percutaneous intervention. It has also been shown that patients with chronic kidney disease who have CK-MB elevation greater than three times the upper normal limit after a successful PCI have a higher incidence of in-hospital complications and a significantly higher mortality rate at 1-year follow-up compared to patients without CK-MB elevation.[19] However, in an interesting analysis by Lindsay et al in patients with normal or mild renal insufficiency (serum creatinine ≤2.0 mg/dl) a postprocedural increase in serum creatinine in the absence of CK-MB elevation was associated with a significant increase in late mortality; of note, however, the converse was not true.[20] A post-PCI increase in CK-MB was not associated with increased 1-year mortality in the absence of a serum creatinine increase. Thus, CIN following PCI was not only a more powerful predictor of late mortality than an increase in CK-MB, but also an independent predictor. Furthermore, the frequency of late adverse events was greatest in patients in whom serum creatinine and CK-MB increased after the procedure. Their rate of either death or myocardial infarction was 26.3%, compared to 7.2% in patients in whom neither was increased (*P*<0.001).

Increased morbidity and mortality in patients who develop CIN was also shown by Rihal et al from the Mayo Clinic.[21] In this study of 7586 patients who underwent PCI, the incidence of CIN (defined as an increase in serum creatinine ≥0.5 mg/dl from baseline) was 3.3%. Patients who developed this complication were older, had a higher incidence of congestive heart failure, hypertension, and diabetes, and were more likely to present with acute myocardial infarction and shock than patients without CIN. According to this study, diabetic patients who had a baseline serum

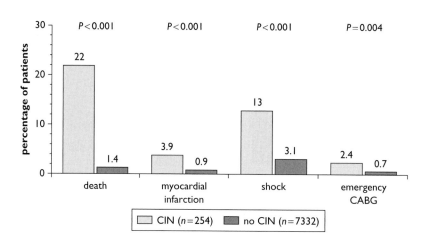

Figure 3.6 *The in-hospital complications of patients who developed contrast-induced nephropathy (CIN) (□) and those who did not (■) in the study by Rihal et al.[21]*

creatinine level < 2.0 mg/dl had a higher risk compared with non-diabetic patients. However, in patients with a serum creatinine > 2 mg/dl, diabetic status did not have an impact, as the rate of CIN was high for both groups. Although the overall incidence of CIN in this study was low, the incidence of in-hospital mortality was 22%, compared to 1.4% in patients who did not develop this complication ($P < 0.0001$) (Figure 3.6). Furthermore, the incidence of in-hospital complications like myocardial infarction, hypotension, shock, hematoma, gastrointestinal bleeding, and emergency coronary artery bypass surgery was significantly higher in patients who developed CIN.[21] Similarly, mortality rate at 1-year follow-up was significantly higher (12.1%) in these patients (non-cumulative).

CIN requiring dialysis

As previously described, CIN requiring dialysis is a rare complication following percutaneous coronary intervention. Nevertheless the consequences are dire, and it is associated with a 6- to 10-fold increase in mortality rates.[1,11,13,15,22] In a retrospective analysis of 7741 patients who underwent PCI at the Washington Hospital Center between January 1994 and July 1998, a total of 51 patients (0.7%) developed CIN that required dialysis replacement therapy.[11] These patients were older, more often female, and had a higher incidence of comorbid conditions such as diabetes, hypertension, and previous coronary artery bypass surgery. Nevertheless, 61% of the patients who required dialysis had a previous history of chronic kidney disease, as defined by a baseline serum creatinine level ≥ 1.8 mg/dl (mean 2.6 ± 1.3 mg/dl) and mean creatinine clearance of 33 ± 17 mg/min. In-hospital mortality rates were significantly higher for patients who required dialysis (27.5% vs 1.0%, $P < 0.0001$). Cardiac death, non-Q-wave myocardial infarction, pulmonary edema, and vascular complications were also significantly increased in these patients (Figure 3.7). The length of stay in the intensive coronary care unit and the average length of stay after the procedure were also significantly longer (18 days vs 4 days, $P < 0.0001$). Of the

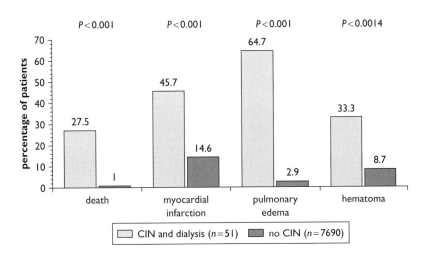

Figure 3.7 *The in-hospital outcomes of patients who developed contrast-induced nephropathy (CIN) that required dialysis replacement therapy (□) and those who did not (■) in the study by Gruberg et al.[11]*

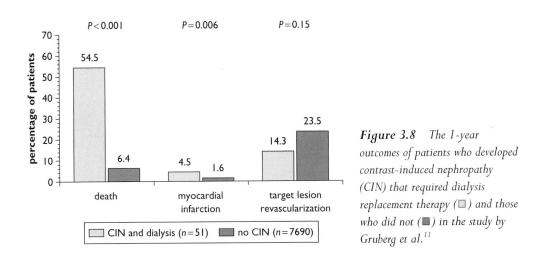

Figure 3.8 *The 1-year outcomes of patients who developed contrast-induced nephropathy (CIN) that required dialysis replacement therapy (□) and those who did not (■) in the study by Gruberg et al.[11]*

51 patients who developed CIN and required dialysis after the procedure, more than half (54.5%) died during the first year (Figure 3.8), while 75% of those discharged on dialysis were on permanent dialysis replacement therapy at 1-year follow-up. These data are consistent with previous observations by McCullough et al,[1] who reported a 35.7% in-hospital mortality rate and 82% mortality at 2-year follow-up in 18 patients who developed CIN and required dialysis.

An analysis from 10 729 procedures from the Blue Cross Blue Shield of Michigan Cardiovascular Consortium registry of PCIs showed that 41 patients (0.44%) developed CIN that

41

required dialysis.[23] These patients were more likely to be female, to have multivessel disease, and to receive non-ionic contrast material. The in-hospital mortality rate was significantly higher for patients who developed CIN that required dialysis compared to those patients who did not (39% vs 1.4%, $P<0.001$). Furthermore, there was a direct relation between the number of risk factors and the occurrence of CIN.

Thus, although CIN that requires dialysis is a rare complication after PCI, it is associated with a poor short- and long-term prognosis. It follows that it is important to identify those patients at the higher risk and use all the necessary precautions to prevent this serious complication.

CIN and acute myocardial infarction

Patients who undergo primary PCI in the acute phase of myocardial infarction may be at a higher risk of developing CIN due to hypotension, the use of large volumes of contrast media, and the fact that starting renal prophylactic measures prior to the procedure is difficult, if not impossible. According to a study by Marenzi and colleagues, 19% of 208 acute myocardial infarction patients who underwent primary PCI developed CIN.[24] However, in those patients with *a priori* reduced renal function (creatinine clearance <60 ml/min), the rate of CIN climbed to 40%. These patients tended to be older and were more likely to have had an anterior wall myocardial infarction, as well as longer time-to-reperfusion and more depressed left ventricular function compared with patients who did not develop CIN. Patients who developed CIN also received a larger volume of contrast material. Remarkably, these patients had a more complicated course during hospitalization, with a high incidence of cardiogenic shock, pulmonary edema, and a significantly higher mortality rate compared with patients who did not develop CIN (31% vs 0.6%, $P<0.0001$) (Figure 3.9). Whether the development of CIN after PCI is just a marker of a severe comorbid state or whether it directly contributes to the poor outcome of these patients has yet to be

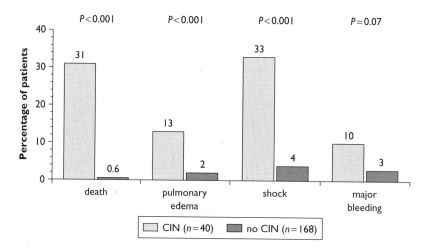

Figure 3.9 *The in-hospital complications of patients who developed contrast-induced nephropathy (CIN) following primary PCI (▢) and those who did not (▢) in the study by Marenzi et al.[24]*

determined. Since the prognosis of these patients is significantly worse, every effort should be made to prevent this complication.

Cardiogenic shock during acute myocardial infarction is associated with very high mortality rates and is the most common cause of death in these patients. Although emergency PCI and revascularization may improve the outcomes of selected cardiogenic shock patients, the impact of CIN in these patients has not been well established. In a retrospective analysis of 118 patients admitted with acute myocardial infarction complicated by cardiogenic shock, acute renal failure occurred in 33% and was associated with a significantly higher in-hospital mortality rate (87%) compared to that observed in patients without acute renal failure (53%).[25] More than half of all patients (56%) underwent acute coronary revascularization. Among those who underwent revascularization and developed acute renal failure, mortality was 85%. In a multiple logistic regression analysis, acute renal failure was the only independent predictor of mortality also in patients who underwent coronary revascularization (OR = 5.7; 95% CI: 1.7–19.5, $P=0.006$).

CIN in the elderly population

As the population ages and interventional physicians become more and more aggressive, the number of elderly patients referred for contrast-based procedures continues to increase. It is well known that elderly patients are at an increased risk of developing CIN, since renal function tends to decrease with age and other risk factors, such as diabetes, congestive heart failure, and dehydration, are more common in these patients. A study by Rich and Crecelius in 203 consecutive patients ≥70 years old undergoing cardiac angiography showed that CIN occurred in 10.5%.[26] In the majority of these patients (57.1%), CIN resolved without further sequelae within 5 to 7 days and in an additional 19% of patients there was partial resolution. Nevertheless, in five patients serum creatinine levels remained significantly elevated at the time of hospital discharge. Three patients (14.3%) who developed this complication died in the course of the hospitalization, none due to causes directly related to CIN but two of them had marked deterioration of renal function, compared to 10 deaths (6.2%) among patients without CIN ($P=$NS).

Conclusion

Despite the fact that numerous preventative methods have been explored to prevent CIN, this complication continues to be a source of concern, particularly in patients with pre-existing renal insufficiency who need to undergo contrast-enhanced radiographic examinations and interventions. In patients with normal renal function, CIN is relatively rare, but its frequency increases in patients with abnormal renal function with or without diabetes mellitus, and all the more in patients with a combination of both diseases. Unfortunately, patients who develop CIN during PCI face a poor prognosis; the condition is associated with increased rates of morbidity and mortality. The length of hospitalization is significantly increased leading to higher utilization of resources and increased hospital costs. CIN requiring dialysis seldom occurs, nevertheless it is an ominous condition associated with high rates of in-hospital complications and mortality rates. Furthermore, more than half of these patients will not survive one year. Therefore, every effort should be made with the ultimate goal of developing new strategies to prevent CIN and its complications.

References

1. McCullough PA, Wolyn R, Rocher LL, Levin RN, O'Neill WW. Acute renal failure after coronary intervention: incidence, risk factors, and relationship to mortality. *Am J Med* 1997; **103**:368–75.
2. Agrawal M, Stouffer GA. Contrast induced nephropathy after angiography. *Am J Med Sci* 2002; **323**:252–8.
3. Calculator available at http://www.kidney.org/professionals/doqi/index.cfm
4. Sarnak MJ, Levey AS, Schoolwerth AC et al. Kidney disease as a risk factor for development of cardiovascular disease. A statement from the American Heart Association Councils on Kidney in Cardiovascular Disease, High Blood Pressure Research, Clinical Cardiology, and Epidemiology and Prevention. *Circulation* 2003; **108**:2154–69.
5. Foley RN, Parfrey PS, Sarnak MJ. Clinical epidemiology of cardiovascular disease in chronic renal disease. *Am J Kidney Dis* 1998; **32**:S112–S119.
6. Porter GA. Contrast-associated nephropathy. *Am J Cardiol* 1989; **64**:22E–26E.
7. Waybill MM, Waybill PN. Contrast media-induced nephrotoxicity: identification of patients at risk and algorithms for prevention. *J Vasc Interven Radiol* 2001; **12**:3–9.
8. Nash K, Hafeez A, Abrinko P, Hou S. Hospital-acquired renal insufficiency. *J Am Soc Nephrol* 1996; **7**:1376.
9. Solomon R. Nephrology forum: contrast-medium-induced acute renal failure. *Kidney Int* 1998; **53**:230–42.
10. Teruel JL, Marcen R, Onaindia JM et al. Renal function impairment caused by intravenous urography: a prospective study. *Arch Intern Med* 1981; **141**:1271–4.
11. Gruberg L, Mehran R, Dangas G et al. Acute renal failure requiring dialysis after percutaneous coronary interventions. *Cathet Cardiovasc Interven* 2001; **52**:409–16.
12. Rudnick MR, Berns JS, Cohen RM, Goldfarb S. Nephrotoxic risks of renal angiography: contrast-media associated nephrotoxicity and atheroembolism – a critical review. *Am J Kidney Dis* 1994; **24**:713–27.
13. Gruberg L, Mintz GS, Dangas G et al. The prognostic implications of further renal function deterioration within 48 h of interventional coronary procedures in patients with pre-existing chronic renal insufficiency. *J Am Coll Cardiol* 2000; **36**:1542–8.
14. Best PJ, Lennon R, Ting HH et al. The impact of renal insufficiency on clinical outcomes in patients undergoing percutaneous coronary interventions. *J Am Coll Cardiol* 2002; **39**:1113–19.
15. Levy EM, Viscoli CM, Horwitz RI. The effect of acute renal failure on mortality. A cohort analysis. *JAMA* 1996; **275**:1489–94.
16. Lindsay J, Apple S, Pinnow EE et al. Percutaneous coronary intervention-associated nephropathy forshadows increased risk of late adverse events in patients with normal baseline serum creatinine. *Cathet Cardiovasc Interven* 2003; **59**:338–43.
17. Gupta R, Gurm HS, Bhatt DL, Chew DP, Ellis SG. Renal failure after percutaneous coronary intervention is associated with high mortality. *Cathet Cardiovasc Interven* 2005; **64**:442–8.
18. Califf RM, Abdelmeguid AE, Kuntz RE et al. Myonecrosis after revascularization procedures. *J Am Coll Cardiol* 1998; **31**:241–51.
19. Gruberg L, Mehran R, Waksman R et al. Creatine kinase-MB fraction elevation after percutaneous coronary intervention in patients with chronic renal failure. *Am J Cardiol* 2001; **87**:1356–60.
20. Lindsay J, Canos DA, Apple S et al. Causes of acute renal dysfunction after percutaneous coronary intervention and comparison of late mortality rates with postprocedure rise of creatinine in kinase-MB versus rise of serum creatinine. *Am J Cardiol* 2004; **94**:786–9.

21. Rihal CS, Textor SC, Grill DE et al. Incidence and prognostic importance of acute renal failure after percutaneous coronary intervention. *Circulation* 2002; **105**:2259–64.

22. Levine GN, Jacobs AK, Keeler GP et al for the CAVEAT-I Investigators. Impact of diabetes mellitus on percutaneous revascularization (CAVEAT-I). *Am J Cardiol* 1997; **79**:748–55.

23. Freeman RV, O'Donnel M, Share D et al for the Blue Cross Shield of Michigan Cardiovascular Consortium (BMC2). Nephropathy requiring dialysis after percutaneous coronary intervention and the critical role of an adjusted contrast dose. *Am J Cardiol* 2002; **90**:1068–73.

24. Marenzi G, Lauri G, Assanelli E et al. Contrast-induced nephropathy in patients undergoing primary angioplasty for acute myocardial infarction. *J Am Coll Cardiol* 2004; **44**:1780–5.

25. Koreny M, Karth GD, Geppert A et al. Prognosis of patients who develop acute renal failure during the first 24 hours of cardiogenic shock after myocardial infarction. *Am J Med* 2002; **112**:115–19.

26. Rich MW, Crecelius CA. Incidence, risk factors, and clinical course of acute renal insufficiency after cardiac catheterization in patients 70 years and older. A prospective study. *Arch Intern Med* 1990; **150**:1237–42.

4. CORONARY RISK AND CHRONIC KIDNEY DISEASE

Rajiv Gupta, Yochai Birnbaum, and
Barry F Uretsky

Introduction

The number of chronic kidney disease (CKD) patients is growing rapidly. In 1998 in the United States alone, 320 000 patients required dialysis, 13.3 million had mild to severe non-dialysis-dependent CKD and another 5.9 million had CKD without decreased glomerular filtration rate (GFR).[1] Coronary artery disease (CAD) has a high prevalence and is the major cause of mortality in CKD patients (Figure 4.1).[2–5] CKD patients also have an increased prevalence of peripheral arterial and cerebrovascular disease, left ventricular hypertrophy, and cardiomyopathy. Whether the increased CAD prevalence in CKD is related to the higher prevalence of traditional risk factors or the presence of risk factors unique to CKD is not totally clear (Table 4.1).[6] A discussion of the relationship of these risk factors to increased coronary events is beyond the scope of this chapter and the reader is directed to recent reviews.[6,7] However, it should be noted that a recent study of 1249 CKD patients has suggested that traditional risk factors are more important as predictors of cardiovascular mortality than the risk factors unique to CKD patients.[8] It is clear, however, that CKD increases the risk of a cardiovascular event and is associated with a worse outcome if it occurs. This chapter will review the increased cardiovascular risk and worsened prognosis associated with renal dysfunction.

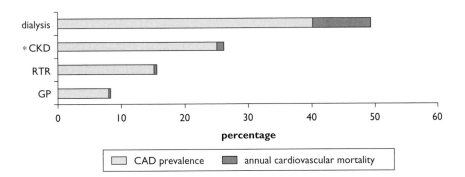

Figure 4.1 *Prevalence of coronary artery disease (CAD) and cardiovascular mortality in chronic kidney disease (CKD) patients. * CKD: mild to moderate chronic kidney disease; prevalence of CAD in this group has been estimated to be intermediate between RTRs and dialysis patients as data are currently unavailable; RTR: renal transplant recipients; GP: general adult population. (Adapted from Gupta et al.[6])*

Table 4.1   Risk factors for coronary artery disease in chronic kidney disease patients

Diabetes	↑ Calcium-phosphate product
Hypertension	Hyperhomocysteinemia
Hyperlipidemia	Oxidative stress
Smoking	CRP, fibrinogen, IL-6, factor VIIc
Positive family history	Hypercoagulability
	Anemia
	Immunosuppressants (RTR)

CRP: C-reactive protein; IL-6: interleukin-6; RTR: renal transplant recipients.
For a full discussion, see reviews by Gupta et al,[6] Yerkey et al,[7] and Shlipak et al.[8]

Definition of renal dysfunction

Serum creatinine (sCr) has been used to estimate glomerular filtration rate (GFR). Use of the Cockroft–Gault equation or the Modification of Diet in Renal Disease study equation (MDRD) to assess renal function provides a more accurate estimate of GFR as it takes the patient's body mass and age into account. Different values have been used by various study groups to define CKD and grade its severity, resulting in difficulty in study comparison. A new classification dividing CKD into five stages depending on estimated GFR may help to facilitate comparison of data from different studies.[6]

Cardiovascular risk associated with renal dysfunction in the community

A decrease in GFR in large population surveys has been associated with increased risk of cardiovascular events. In a diverse population of 1 120 295 adults in the Kaiser Permanente Renal Registry with a median follow-up of 2.8 years, the adjusted risk of all-cause mortality and cardiovascular events (hospitalization for CAD events, heart failure, stroke, or peripheral arterial disease) increased as GFR decreased below 60 ml/min per $1.73\,m^2$ body surface area (adjusted hazard ratio for death 1.2 for GFR = 45–59 ml/min, 1.8 for GFR = 30–45 ml/min, 3.2 for GFR = 15–29 ml/min, and 5.9 for GFR < 15 ml/min) (Figure 4.2).[9]

In a long-term follow-up of CKD patients undergoing coronary angiography, the hazard ratio for subsequent acute myocardial infarction (AMI) or death was 2.3 for GFR < 60 ml/min and 5.1 for GFR < 30 ml/min.[10] Even CKD patients with 'normal' angiography demonstrated an increased risk of AMI (5.2% vs 0.7% in non-CKD patients, $P = 0.01$) and mortality (24.7% vs 3.9%, $P < 0.001$).

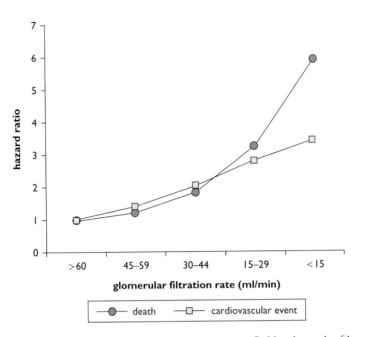

Figure 4.2 *Hazard ratio for death and cardiovascular events stratified by glomerular filtration rate. (Adapted from Go et al.[9])*

Cardiovascular risk in renal patients with acute coronary syndromes

The outcomes of renal patients with AMI have been dismal. Some studies have focused on ST segment elevation MI (STEMI) exclusively, whereas others have included patients with both STEMI and non-STEMI.

The prognosis in STEMI treated with thrombolysis as well as non-STEMI worsens as the GFR declines. A meta-analysis of STEMI thrombolytic trials showed an inverse correlation between 30-day mortality and renal function.[11] A retrospective analysis of CKD patients with STEMI showed a lower 30-day mortality with thrombolysis (8.3%) than percutaneous coronary intervention (PCI) (37.1%, $P=0.04$), emphasizing the current uncertainty of the preferred treatment for STEMI in CKD patients.[12]

CKD appears to adversely affect AMI prognosis irrespective of the ST segment status. In a large substudy of four trials of mild to moderate CKD patients with both STEMI and non-ST segment elevation ACS, patients with CKD had higher mortality at 30 days and 6 months than non-CKD patients regardless of ST segment status.[13] A study of 3106 AMI (both STEMI and non-STEMI) patients showed an in-hospital mortality of 2% in normal renal function compared with 6% with mild CKD (creatinine clearance (CCr) = 51–75 ml/min), 14% with moderate CKD (CCr 35–50 ml/min), 21% with severe CKD (CCr < 35 ml/min), and 30% in dialysis patients, ($P<0.001$) (Figure 4.3).[5] The 1-year mortality after AMI (both STEMI and non-STEMI) appears to be higher in dialysis

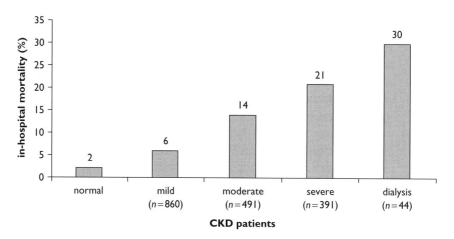

Figure 4.3 *In-hospital mortality after acute myocardial infarction. See text for details. CKD: chronic kidney disease. (Adapted from Wright et al.[5])*

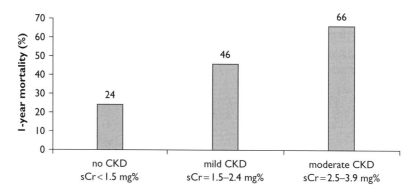

Figure 4.4 *One-year mortality after acute myocardial infarction in patients older than 64 years. CKD: chronic kidney disease; sCr: serum creatinine. (Adapted from Shlipak et al.[15])*

patients compared with renal transplant recipients (RTRs) (59% versus 24%).[14] In a post-AMI (both STEMI and non-STEMI) Medicare cohort comprising 130 099 patients, 1-year mortality was 24% without CKD, 46% with mild CKD (sCr 1.5–2.4 mg/dl), and 66% with moderate CKD (sCr 2.5–3.9 mg/dl) ($P < 0.001$) (Figure 4.4).[15] In a substudy of the Valsartan in Acute Myocardial Infarction Trial (VALIANT) involving 14 527 patients with mild CKD (sCr < 2.5 mg/dl) and AMI (both Q and non-Q AMI) complicated by clinical or radiologic signs of heart failure or systolic dysfunction, or both, patients were grouped according to estimated GFR using the MDRD equation.[16] Each reduction of the estimated GFR by 10 units below 81.0 ml/min per 1.73 m^2 was associated with a hazard ratio of 1.10 (95% confidence interval 1.08–1.12), for the risk of death or composite endpoint (cardiovascular death, reinfarction, congestive heart failure, stroke, or resuscitation after cardiac arrest).[16]

The increase in mortality risk with worsening renal function is seen not only in AMI but also in unstable angina.[17] Patients with mild to moderate CKD and non-ST segment elevation ACS in the PRISM-PLUS (Platelet Receptor Inhibition in Ischemic Syndrome Management in Patients Limited by Unstable Signs and Symptoms) trial showed an increased risk of death/non-fatal myocardial infarction at 48 hours, 7 days, 30 days, and 6 months with decreasing creatinine clearance.[18]

Cardiovascular risk with medical therapy

Aspirin, beta-blockers, and statins appear to be underused in patients with reduced GFR, which may account in part for an increase in long-term mortality.[16] Also, utilization of diagnostic coronary angiography, PCI, and glycoprotein IIb/IIIa antagonists decreases as the renal function declines. Data on toxicities of cardiovascular drugs such as glycoprotein IIb/IIIa antagonists and their effects on 'hard' outcomes are currently limited as these patients have been excluded from randomized trials. In 310 patients with CCr <60 ml/min increased major bleeding events were noted with glycoprotein IIb/IIIa antagonist use and worsening CCr in non-dialysis CKD patients. However, an overall protective effect on in-hospital mortality was seen with glycoprotein IIb/IIIa antagonist use.[19] Direct thrombin inhibitors undergo renal clearance and should be used cautiously until more data are available. Bivalirudin may be equally or more effective than unfractionated heparin, with lesser bleeding according to a meta-analysis.[20] Low molecular weight heparin may accumulate in renal failure and, in the absence of more data, unfractionated heparin is preferred.

Concern regarding increased bleeding risk, hyperkalemia, worsening of renal failure, dose adjustment, and special precautions for a number of cardiovascular drugs limits their use in CKD patients.[6]

Cardiovascular risk after PCI in CKD

Early small studies using balloon angioplasty in hemodialysis (HD) patients have shown an initial angiographic success of 56–96% with high restenosis rates (60–81%).[21] Lower restenosis rates (30%) were observed in later studies.[22] Dialysis-dependence alone or in combination with diabetes is an independent predictor of cardiac death and non-fatal myocardial infarction after PCI.[23] Primary angioplasty in AMI (55% stent use) showed a higher 30-day death rate in CKD (7.5%) versus non-CKD patients (0.8%, $P<0.0001$) with a similar trend at 1 year.[24] In multivariable analysis, CKD had the highest RR (5.7) for mortality of all factors studied. CKD patients undergoing saphenous vein graft interventions also show a higher in-hospital and 1-year mortality compared with non-CKD patients.[25]

Most studies in CKD patients have shown a paradox of higher long-term mortality without a difference in target lesion revascularization (TLR) or restenosis compared with non-CKD patients. In a study utilizing only balloon angioplasty, a higher in-hospital and 1-year mortality rate was observed without a difference in TLR in dialysis and non-dialysis CKD compared with non-CKD patients (Figure 4.5).[22] In studies with increased stent use (40%), mortality has been higher in dialysis versus non-CKD patients (11% versus 2%, $P<0.03$) without a difference in restenosis.[26]

51

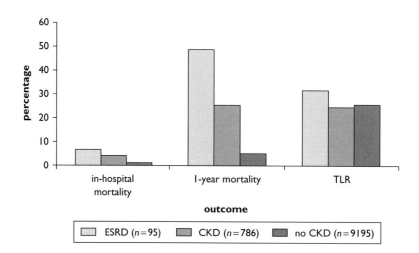

Figure 4.5 *Mortality and target lesion revascularization (TLR) after PCI in CKD versus non-CKD patients. CKD: chronic kidney disease; ESRD: end-stage renal disease; PCI: percutaneous coronary intervention. (Adapted from Gruberg et al.[22])*

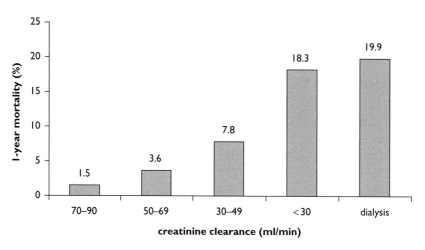

Figure 4.6 *One-year mortality after PCI in patients stratified by creatinine clearance. (Adapted from Best et al.[27])*

In 5327 post-PCI patients (68% stents), 1-year mortality was 1.5% (RR 1.5) with CCr 70–90 ml/min, 3.6% (RR 2.3) with CCr 50–69 ml/min, 7.8% (RR 3.7) with CCr 30–49 ml/min, 18.3% with CCr < 30 ml/min, and 19.9% (RR 8.9) in dialysis patients (P = 0.001) (Figure 4.6).[27] Again, no difference in the TLR was noted between the CCr subgroups. In a substudy of 848 patients with STEMI (58% stents, SCr < 2.7 mg/dl) in the Stent Primary Angioplasty in Myocardial Infarction (Stent-PAMI) trial, patients with CCr < 75 ml/min had a 9.3% incidence of death versus 1.7% with CCr > 75 ml/min (P < 0.0001) and a 25% incidence of major adverse cardiovascular events (death, non-fatal reinfarction, disabling stroke, and ischemia-driven target vessel revascularization) versus 19% with CCr >75 ml/min (P=0.03) after 1 year.[28] However, there was no difference in TLR between the treatment groups. In 11 187 patients with sCr < 1.8 mg/dl (grouped by estimated CCr < 60, 60–89, > 89 ml/min) from the PRESTO trial (Prevention of Restenosis with Tranilast and its Outcomes), there was no increase after bare metal stenting in restenosis or target vessel revascularization at 9-month angiographic follow-up.[29] A mild increase in mortality was found in the patients with the lowest CCr, but it was not significant after adjustment was made for confounding variables. These data suggest that CKD *per se* does not affect the clinical or angiographic restenosis rate or TLR. The explanation of increased mortality after PCI in CKD appears to be multifactorial. CKD patients as a group are older, are more frequently females, have a lower left ventricular ejection fraction, increased prevalence of left ventricular hypertrophy, a higher incidence of triple vessel coronary artery disease, and increased comorbidities such as cerebrovascular disease, peripheral vascular disease, diabetes, and hypertension. CKD patients also receive optimal medical therapy less frequently including reperfusion, aspirin, and beta-blockers. These factors may explain the high mortality in the absence of increased restenosis or TLR.

Multivessel stenting may be a therapeutic option in CKD patients. In a substudy of 290 CKD patients (CCr < 60 ml/min) in the Arterial Revascularization Therapies Study (ARTS), there was no difference in the composite of death, myocardial infarction, or stroke between multivessel bare-metal stenting and coronary artery bypass graft surgery (CABG). CABG showed a reduced risk for repeat revascularization (HR (hazard ratio) = 0.28; 95% CI 0.14–0.54; P<0.01). CKD was associated with a nearly 2-fold increased risk for the composite outcome compared with normal renal function, which remained significant after multivariate adjustment.[30]

Data on the use of drug-eluting stents in CKD are currently unavailable and eagerly awaited.

Cardiovascular risk after CABG in CKD

CABG in dialysis patients has a perioperative mortality of approximately 7–10%, which is at least 3 to 4 times higher than non-CKD patients, and 5-year mortality is estimated at 48% versus 15% in non-CKD patients (Figure 4.7).[6] Most studies are retrospective, unadjusted for comorbidities, and have a small sample size. In studies with adjustment, CKD remains a highly significant predictor for decreased long-term survival.[31] Not unexpectedly, hemodialysis-dependent diabetics suffer worse long-term outcomes after CABG than non-diabetics.[32]

Limited data on CABG outcomes in mild or moderate CKD patients show worsened short- and long-term prognosis. CKD patients (vs non-CKD patients) have longer in-hospital and intensive care unit stay and more frequent postoperative dialysis.[33] In a prospective 1427-patient study, sCr ≥ 1.5 mg/dl increased the length of hospital stay and the need for postoperative dialysis.[34] In-hospital mortality increased with a rise in preoperative sCr (2.3%, sCr < 1.5 mg/dl; 18.5%, sCr ≥ 1.7 mg/dl). In a prospective study of 2222 mild CKD patients, 7.7% had postoperative renal dysfunction associated with prolonged intensive care unit and hospital stays and increased mortality.[35]

Long-term outcomes in the Bypass Angioplasty Revascularization Investigation (BARI) showed a higher risk of all-cause (RR 2.2) and cardiac (RR 2.8) deaths and increased cardiac admissions in CKD patients who underwent CABG or PCI, with a 7-year mortality of 70% in patients with

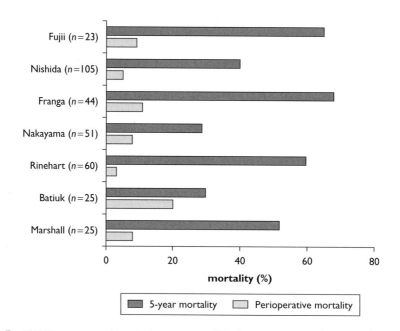

Figure 4.7 *CABG outcomes in hemodialysis patients. CABG: coronary artery bypass grafting. (Adapted from Gupta et al.[6])*

CKD and DM.[36] In another analysis of mild to moderate CKD patients, in-hospital CABG mortality was 11% and actuarial survival at 10 years was 32%, similar to dialysis patients.[37]

There have been very few studies addressing CABG outcomes in RTRs. In a study of 131 RTRs, there was a perioperative mortality of 3.2%, with no deaths during 5 year follow-up.[38] In 45 RTRs undergoing PCI or CABG, actuarial survival at 1, 3, and 5 years was 93%, 78%, and 60%.[39]

Conclusions

CKD is increasing to epidemic proportions. It is associated with increased risk of cardiovascular events and worsened prognosis across the entire spectrum of the disease and revascularization strategies. Despite the obvious impact of CAD on the natural history of CKD, there is paucity of data and an urgent need for randomized trials for an evidence-based approach to management.

References

1. Sarnak MJ, Levey AS, Schoolwerth AC et al. Kidney disease as a risk factor for development of cardiovascular disease. *Circulation* 2003; **108**:2154–69.
2. Foley RN, Parfrey PS, Sarnak MJ. Clinical epidemiology of cardiovascular disease in chronic renal disease. *Am J Kidney Dis* 1998; **32(Suppl 3)**:112–19.
3. US Renal Data System 1992, Annual Report IV. Comorbid conditions and correlations with mortality risk among 3,399 incident hemodialysis patients. *Am J Kidney Dis* 1992; **20(Suppl 2)**:32–8.

4. US Renal Data System 1997, Annual Data Report. Bethesda, MD, 1997.

5. Wright RS, Reeder GS, Herzog CA et al. Acute myocardial infarction and renal dysfunction: a high-risk combination. *Ann Intern Med* 2002; **137**:563–70.

6. Gupta R, Birnbaum Y, Uretsky BF. The renal patient with coronary artery disease: current concepts and dilemmas. *J Am Coll Cardiol* 2004; **44**:1343–53.

7. Yerkey MW, Kernis SJ, Franklin BA, Sandberg KR, McCullough PA. Renal dysfunction and acceleration of coronary disease. *Heart* 2004; **90**:961–6.

8. Shlipak MG, Fried LF, Cushman M et al. Cardiovascular mortality risk in chronic kidney disease: comparison of traditional and novel risk factors. *JAMA* 2005; **292**:1737–45.

9. Go AS, Chertow GM, Fan D, McCulloch CE, Hsu C. Chronic kidney disease and risks of death, cardiovascular events, and hospitalization. *N Engl J Med* 2004; **351**:1296–305.

10. Zebrack JS, Anderson JL, Beddhu S et al. Do associations with C-reactive protein and extent of coronary disease account for the increased cardiovascular risk of renal insufficiency? *J Am Coll Cardiol* 2003; **42**:57–63.

11. Gibson CM, Pinto SD, Murphy SA et al. Association of creatinine and creatinine clearance in acute myocardial infarction with subsequent mortality. *J Am Coll Cardiol* 2003; **42**:1535–43.

12. Dragu R, Behar S, Boyko V et al. Should primary percutaneous coronary intervention be the preferred method of myocardial perfusion for ST elevation acute coronary syndromes in patients with renal failure? *Circulation* 2003; **108**:Suppl IV–614.

13. Al Suwaidi J, Reddan DN, Williams K et al. Prognostic implications of abnormalities in renal function in patients with acute coronary syndromes. *Circulation* 2002; **106**:974–80.

14. Herzog CA, Ma JZ, Collins AJ. Poor long-term survival after acute myocardial infarction among patients on long-term dialysis. *N Engl J Med* 1998; **339**:799–805.

15. Shlipak MG, Heidenreich PA, Noguchi H et al. Association of renal insufficiency with treatment and outcomes after myocardial infarction in elderly patients. *Ann Intern Med* 2002; **37**:555–62.

16. Anavekar NS, McMurray JJV, Velazquez EJ et al. Relation between renal dysfunction and cardiovascular outcomes after myocardial infarction. *N Engl J Med* 2004; **351**:1285–95.

17. Masoudi FA, Plomondon ME, Magid DJ, Sales A, Rumsfeld JS. Renal insufficiency and mortality from acute coronary syndromes. *Am Heart J* 2004; **147**:623–9.

18. Januzzi JL, Snapinn SM, DiBattiste PM, Jang IK, Theroux P. Benefits and safety of tirofiban among acute coronary syndrome patients with mild to moderate renal insufficiency. *Circulation* 2002; **105**:2361–6.

19. Freeman RV, Mehta RH, Al Badr W et al. Influence of concurrent renal dysfunction on outcomes of patients with acute coronary syndromes and implications of the use of glycoprotein IIb/IIIa inhibitors. *J Am Coll Cardiol* 2003; **41**:718–24.

20. Chew DP, Bhatt DL, Kimball W et al. Bivalirudin produces increasing benefit with decreasing renal function: a meta-analysis of randomized trials. *Am J Cardiol* 2003; **92**:919–23.

21. Schoebel FC, Gradaus F, Ivens K et al. Restenosis after elective coronary balloon angioplasty in patients with end stage renal disease: a case control study using quantitative coronary angiography. *Heart* 1997; **78**:337–342.

22. Gruberg L, Dangas G, Mehran R et al. Clinical outcome following percutaneous coronary interventions in patients with chronic renal failure. *Cathet Cardiovasc Interv* 2002; **55**:66–72.

23. Le Feuvre C, Borentain M, Beygui F et al. Comparison of short and long-term outcomes of coronary angioplasty in patients with and without diabetes mellitus and with and without hemodialysis. *Am J Cardiol* 2003; **92**:721–5.

24. Sadeghi HM, Stone GW, Grines CL et al. Impact of renal insufficiency in patients undergoing primary angioplasty for acute myocardial infarction. *Circulation* 2003; **108**:2769–75.

25. Gruberg L, Weissman NJ, Pichard AD et al. Impact of renal function on morbidity and mortality after percutaneous aortocoronary saphenous vein graft intervention. *Am Heart J* 2003; **145**:529–34.

26. Le Feuvre C, Dambrin G, Helft G et al. Clinical outcome following coronary angioplasty in dialysis patients: a case control study in the era of coronary stenting. *Heart* 2001; **85**:556–60.

27. Best PJM, Lennon R, Ting HH et al. The impact of renal insufficiency on clinical outcomes in patients undergoing percutaneous coronary interventions. *J Am Coll Cardiol* 2002; **39**:1113–19.

28. Dixon SR, O'Neill WW, Sadeghi HM et al. Usefulness of creatinine clearance in predicting early and late death after primary angioplasty for acute myocardial infarction. *Am J Cardiol* 2003; **91**:1454–7.

29. Best PJM, Berger PB, Davis BR et al. Impact of mild or moderate chronic kidney disease on the frequency of restenosis: results from the PRESTO trial. *J Am Coll Cardiol* 2004; **44**:1786–91.

30. Ix JH, Mercado N, Shlipak MG et al. Association of chronic kidney disease with clinical outcomes after coronary revascularization: the Arterial Revascularization Therapies Study (ARTS). *Am Heart J* 2005; **149**:512–19.

31. Dacey LJ, Liu JY, Braxton JH et al. Long-term survival of dialysis patients after coronary bypass grafting. *Ann Thorac Surg* 2002; **74**:458–63.

32. Hosoda Y, Yamamoto T, Takazawa K et al. Coronary artery bypass grafting in patients on chronic hemodialysis: surgical outcome in diabetic nephropathy versus nondiabetic nephropathy patients. *Ann Thorac Surg* 2001; **71**:543–8.

33. Rao V, Weisel RD, Buth KJ et al. Coronary artery bypass grafting in patients with non-dialysis-dependent renal insufficiency. *Circulation* 1997; **96(Suppl 2)**:38–45.

34. Weerasinghe A, Hornick P, Smith P, Taylor K, Ratnatunga C. Coronary artery bypass grafting in non-dialysis-dependent mild to moderate renal dysfunction. *J Thorac Cardiovasc Surg* 2001; **121**:1083–9.

35. Mangano CM, Diamondstone LS, Ramsay JG et al. Renal dysfunction after myocardial revascularization: risk factors, adverse outcomes, and hospital resource utilization. *Ann Intern Med* 1998; **128**:194–203.

36. Bypass Angioplasty Revascularization Investigation (BARI) Investigators, Szczech LA, Best PJ, Crowley E et al. Outcomes of patients with chronic renal insufficiency in BARI. *Circulation* 2002; **105**:2253–8.

37. Nakayama Y, Sakata R, Ura M, Itoh T. Long-term results of coronary artery bypass grafting in patients with renal insufficiency. *Ann Thorac Surg* 2003; **75**:496–500.

38. Dresler C, Uthoff K, Wahlers T et al. Open heart operations after renal transplantation. *Ann Thorac Surg* 1997; **63**:143–6.

39. Ferguson ER, Hudson SL, Diethelm AG et al. Outcome after myocardial revascularization and renal transplantation. *Ann Surg* 1999; **230**:232–41.

5. EFFECTS OF CHRONIC KIDNEY DISEASE AND CONTRAST-INDUCED NEPHROPATHY ON PROGNOSIS AND TREATMENT OUTCOMES OF ACUTE CORONARY SYNDROMES

Giancarlo Marenzi and Antonio L Bartorelli

There is increasing evidence that chronic kidney disease (CKD) is associated with accelerated atherogenesis, and that any degree of renal insufficiency is an independent risk factor for increased cardiovascular events and portends a worsened prognosis in patients with coronary artery disease.[1,2] More recently, the pervasive adverse influence of renal insufficiency has also been demonstrated in the setting of acute coronary syndromes (ACS). Among ACS patients, CKD doubles mortality rates and is third only to cardiogenic shock and congestive heart failure as a predictor of mortality.[3] Antithrombotic agents and percutaneous coronary intervention (PCI) are clearly emerging as the cornerstones of treatment patterns in patients presenting with ACS. However, despite the increasing number of CKD patients with a broad range of ACS at presentation, evidence-based data with established or newer drugs and interventional strategies are still lacking in this population. Ideally, these are the patients to whom recent therapeutic advances should be aggressively applied, in order to minimize their increased risk. Ironically, although they may derive the greatest benefit from proven therapies, application of strategies for reducing their cardiovascular morbidity and mortality seems to be limited when compared to patients with normal renal function. The almost uniform exclusion of patients with CKD from randomized studies evaluating new targeted therapies for ACS, and concern about further deterioration of renal function and therapy-related toxic effects, may explain the apparent reluctance of physicians to use these treatments in patients with renal insufficiency. The paradoxic pattern of undertreatment in this subgroup of high-risk patients could, however, contribute to their excessive mortality. As French and Wright pointed out, the time has come to move beyond the attitude of 'therapeutic nihilism' toward patients with renal failure, and develop targeted strategies from well-designed research which will ultimately reduce the burden of risk in this population and achieve improved outcomes.[4]

This chapter reviews the clinical and prognostic relevance of renal insufficiency, as well as that of contrast-induced nephropathy (CIN) in ACS patients, with reference to unresolved issues and uncertainties regarding recommended medical therapies and interventional strategies. Given the different prognosis and treatment modalities in patients with ST-segment elevation myocardial infarction (STEMI) and in those with non-ST-segment elevation acute coronary syndrome (NSTE-ACS), such as unstable angina and non-ST-elevation myocardial infarction, the two clinical conditions will be considered separately.

Prognostic relevance of chronic kidney disease in acute coronary syndromes

ST-segment elevation myocardial infarction

The fundamental work of Herzog et al[5] was the initial observation that revealed the poor prognosis faced by patients with endstage renal disease (ESRD) who suffer from acute myocardial infarction (AMI). Using the US Renal Data System data base, the investigators examined the outcome of 34 189 patients on long-term dialysis after a first episode of AMI, and documented an in-hospital mortality of 26% and a dismal long-term survival. The 1-year and 2-year mortality rates for the entire cohort were 59% and 73%, respectively. It is noteworthy that most patients on dialysis, who had AMI, died of heart disease. These observations were confirmed by Chertow et al,[6] who reported a 30-day mortality rate of 20% and a 1-year mortality rate of 53%, after AMI, in 640 patients with ESRD. Interestingly, 88% of the patients were treated with pharmacologic therapy alone, 7% with PCI, and 5% with coronary artery bypass grafting (CABG). Multivariate analysis showed only a trend toward a reduced risk of death in patients who underwent surgical revascularization. Thus, it is not possible to determine from this study whether percutaneous or surgical interventions are clearly superior or not to medical therapy alone in patients with ESRD after AMI. Beattie et al[7] extended the investigation to patients with advanced renal dysfunction who were not on dialysis therapy. They analyzed a prospective coronary care unit registry of 1724 patients with STEMI admitted over an 8-year period at a single tertiary-care center. Patients were stratified into groups based on different corrected creatinine clearance (CrCl) values. A graded rise in in-hospital complications and death rate, as well as a reduction in long-term survival, were observed across increasing renal dysfunction strata. This study, as well as another by McCullough et al,[8] showed a similar graded increase in the relative risk of atrial and ventricular arrhythmias, heart block, asystole, pulmonary congestion, and cardiogenic shock in parallel with progressive renal impairment. Moreover, the use of mortality-reducing treatments, including primary angioplasty, thrombolysis, and beta-blockers, decreased with the progressive decline of renal function, suggesting a treatment bias in favor of patients with less advanced renal dysfunction (Figure 5.1). While the lower rates of PCI may be rationally explained by the fear of an increased risk of CIN and of the associated high mortality rate, the potential risk of bleeding and hemodynamic complications constitutes only a partial justification for the less frequent use of thrombolysis and beta-blockers.

More recently, two large studies revealed the significant morbidity and mortality risk faced by patients with even minor renal insufficiency who are admitted with STEMI. Wright et al[9] examined treatment patterns, in-hospital complications, and short- and long-term survival in 3106 patients with STEMI in relation to their renal function. CrCl values, derived by the Cockcroft–Gault formula from serum creatinine (sCr) concentration,[10] were used to stratify patients into five groups: normal renal function (CrCl > 75 ml/min), mild renal insufficiency (CrCl > 50 and ≤ 75 ml/min), moderate renal insufficiency (CrCl ≥ 35 and ≤ 50 ml/min), severe renal insufficiency (CrCl < 35 ml/min), and ESRD, defined as treatment with renal replacement therapy for at least 1 month before admission. They observed a gradient of increased risk of death in all groups of patients with renal dysfunction, even in those with mild renal insufficiency: in-hospital mortality

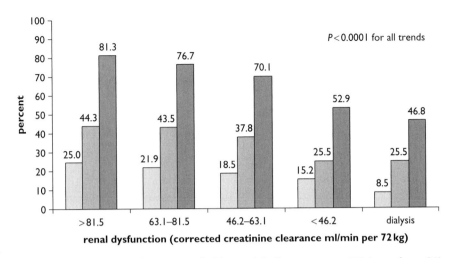

Figure 5.1 *Treatment received for AMI stratified by renal dysfunction group. (▢) Angioplasty; (▨) thrombolysis; (▪) beta-blockers. (From Beattie et al.[7])*

was 2% in patients with normal renal function and progressively increased to 6%, 14%, 21%, and 30% in parallel with renal function worsening. Patients with renal dysfunction also developed more AMI-related complications, including atrial fibrillation, congestive heart failure, and mechanical complications. Reperfusion therapy (intravenous fibrinolysis or primary PCI) was used less frequently (24%) in patients with any degree of renal dysfunction than in patients without renal insufficiency, and was associated with improved long-term survival, but did not reduce the risk of in-hospital mortality. Similarly, the use of aspirin, beta-blockers and intravenous heparin during the first 24 hours of hospitalization was less frequent in patients with ESRD and moderate-to-severe renal insufficiency; these trends persisted with therapies prescribed at hospital discharge, including ACE-inhibitors and beta-blockers. Thus, this study confirms previous observations in CKD patients with STEMI, and suggests gradients of increased risk and less aggressive care that parallel the degree of renal dysfunction. However, the increased postdischarge survival, observed when more aggressive therapies were used, underscores the importance of improving the treatment approach in these patients.

Similar findings were also reported by Shlipak et al[11] in 130 099 elderly patients (age ≥ 65 years) with AMI (about 30% of whom had STEMI). In this large cohort study, mild renal insufficiency was defined as an sCr level between 1.5 and 2.4 mg/dl (28.3% of the study population), and moderate renal insufficiency as an sCr level between 2.5 and 3.9 mg/dl (8.4%). Patients with severe renal insufficiency (sCr ≥ 4.0 mg/dl) were excluded from the analysis. Renal dysfunction turned out to be strongly associated with survival after AMI in elderly patients (Figure 5.2). In particular, one month after hospital admission, mortality for patients with moderate renal insufficiency was 44%, compared with 13% for patients who had relatively normal renal function. Furthermore, the study demonstrated that patients with normal renal function were treated with aspirin and beta-blockers 20% more often and were more than twice as likely to receive thrombolytic therapy, coronary angiography, and angioplasty as patients with moderate renal insufficiency. Among patients

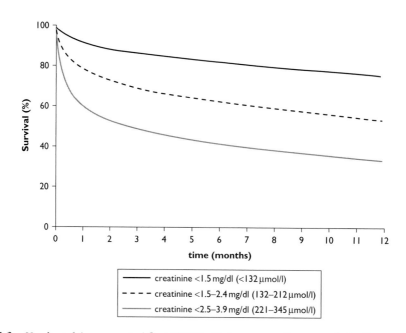

Figure 5.2 *Unadjusted 1-year survival for 130 099 elderly patients after myocardial infarction, by initial serum creatinine levels. (From Shlipak MG et al.[11] From* Annals of Internal Medicine, *with permission.)*

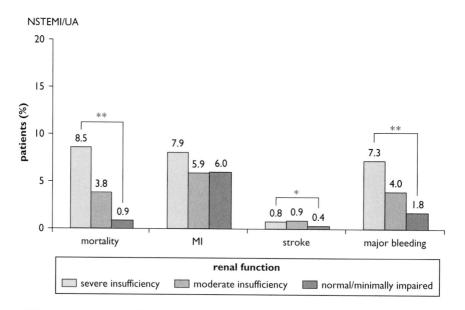

Figure 5.3 *Hospital outcomes for patients with non-ST-segment elevation myocardial infarction/unstable angina (NSTEMI/UA). *P <0.05 across all categories of renal function; **P <0.0001 across all categories of renal function. (Modified from Santopinto et al.[16])*

surviving up to hospital discharge, those with no renal insufficiency were most likely to be prescribed aspirin and beta-blockers, those with mild renal insufficiency most often received ACE inhibitors, and those with moderate renal insufficiency most often received calcium channel blockers. All these studies, as well as a Danish study evaluating 6252 patients included in the TRAndopril Cardiac Evaluation (TRACE) register,[12] support the evidence of a strikingly high mortality after STEMI among patients with renal insufficiency. Moreover, they demonstrate that beneficial therapies, such as aspirin, beta-blockers, and ACE inhibitors, are underutilized despite increased prevalence of hypertension, congestive heart failure, and coronary artery disease, and despite the fact that these medications are associated with a substantial survival benefit in patients with normal renal function. In addition, this 'therapeutic nihilism' is in marked contrast to the results of previous studies demonstrating that ACE inhibitors and beta-blockers are associated with more beneficial effects in patients with renal insufficiency than in patients with preserved renal function.[13,14] Nevertheless, the results of the Valsartan in Acute Myocardial Infarction Trial (VALIANT) suggest that the outcome of CKD patients remains worse, even if a more aggressive therapeutic approach is applied.[15] This trial examined 14 527 patients and found that pre-existing renal insufficiency was a significant independent risk factor for adverse events in patients who had AMI complicated by heart failure, left ventricular systolic dysfunction, or both, despite an apparent optimal postdischarge treatment (all patients received valsartan, captopril, or a combination of both). Unadjusted estimates of 3-year mortality progressively increased in parallel with reduction in renal function of up to 45.5% for patients with an estimated glomerular filtration rate (GFR) of less than 45 ml/min per 1.73 m^2. As patients with a baseline sCr > 2.5 mg/dl were excluded from the study, it is reasonable to suppose that, for patients with a more compromised renal function, a lower survival rate may be expected. These results suggest that even appropriate postdischarge therapy, given in a timely manner, may not be sufficient to improve post-AMI outcome in this population. However, it may also be postulated that, if less than appropriate therapy were provided, even worse outcomes could be expected, and that more aggressive treatment of AMI and primary and secondary prevention, specifically targeted to these high-risk patients, are the only effective strategies for reducing the overall disease burden.

Non-ST-segment elevation acute coronary syndromes

Several observational studies have found that, in the setting of NSTE-ACS, in-hospital outcomes and mid- to long-term mortality are worse among patients with renal insufficiency.[16-18] It has been suggested that CKD be considered a risk factor, and that measurement of renal function be included as an additional and important element in the risk stratification process of patients presenting with ACS.

The Global Registry of Acute Coronary Events (GRACE), a large prospective multinational registry, including the full spectrum of patients with ACS, evaluated the prognostic impact of sCr levels on hospital mortality and adverse outcomes in 11 774 patients (60% of whom had NSTE-ACS).[16] Patients were divided into three groups according to their CrCl values: > 60 ml/min or normal renal function (including patients with minimally impaired renal function); 30–60 ml/min or moderate renal insufficiency, and < 30 ml/min or severe renal insufficiency. In comparison with patients with normal or minimally impaired renal function, patients with moderate and severe renal insufficiency were at a significantly increased risk of hospital mortality and major bleeding episodes. Worse hospital outcomes were observed for all study patients with a diagnosis of ACS at admission, including the subgroup with NSTE-ACS (Figure 5.3). Other studies have definitely confirmed the close association between renal insufficiency and increased risk of death in patients with NSTE-ACS at presentation.[19–23] The significant contribution of renal function evaluation to risk stratification was recently demonstrated by Gibson et al,[24] who pooled data from five international multicenter trials (TIMI 11A and B, TIMI 12, OPUS-TIMI 16, and TACTICS-TIMI 18) and analyzed 13 307 patients with NSTE-ACS. Notably, these trials excluded patients with an sCr level above 2.0 mg/dl, 2.0 mg/dl, 1.5 mg/dl, 1.6 mg/dl, and 2.5 mg/dl, respectively. As a consequence, moderate to severe renal insufficiency (GFR < 60 ml/min per 1.73 m^2) was present in 15.7% of patients, while only 0.67% of the patients had a GFR < 30 ml/min per 1.73 m^2. In this study, a significant and graded association was observed between reduced GFR and 30-day and 6-month mortality: 1.3% and 2.5% for patients with normal renal function, 2.1% and 3.8% for patients with mild renal insufficiency, and 5% and 9.5% for patients with moderate to severe renal insufficiency, respectively (P for trend < 0.001). In parallel, there was a stepwise increase in the incidence of stroke, major bleeding, recurrent myocardial infarction, and recurrent ischemia with worsening GFR (Figure 5.4). Interestingly, within each GFR category, high Thrombolysis in Myocardial Infarction (TIMI) risk scores and augmented levels of biomarkers (C-reactive protein, B-type natriuretic peptide, and troponin I) were associated with a significant increase in mortality as compared with low TIMI scores and normal levels of biomarkers (Figure 5.5), demonstrating the prognostic value of GFR in addition to the traditional clinical risk stratification of patients with NSTE-ACS.

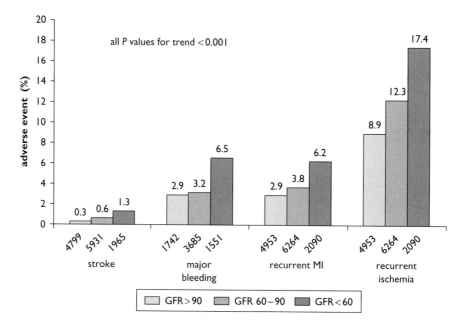

Figure 5.4   *Incidence of adverse event by glomerular filtration rate (GFR) groups: stroke, in-hospital TIMI major bleeding, recurrent myocardial infarction (MI), and recurrent ischemia at 30 days. The number of patients within each subgroup is displayed at the bottom of each bar. GFR is expressed in ml/min per 1.73 m^2. (From Gibson et al.[24])*

(a) *P* value for trend = 0.007 between GFR groups with hs-CRP < 1.5 mg/dl
    P value for trend = 0.001 between GFR groups with hs-CRP ≥ 1.5 mg/dl
    *P < 0.001

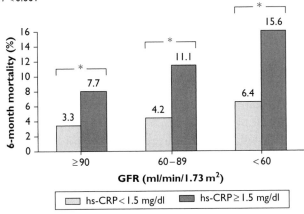

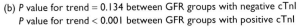

(b) *P* value for trend = 0.134 between GFR groups with negative cTnl
    P value for trend < 0.001 between GFR groups with positive cTnl

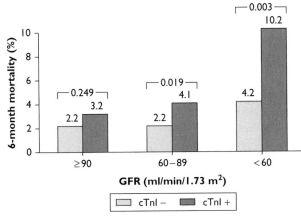

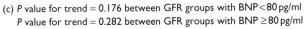

(c) *P* value for trend = 0.176 between GFR groups with BNP < 80 pg/ml
    P value for trend = 0.282 between GFR groups with BNP ≥ 80 pg/ml

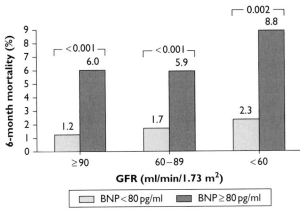

Figure 5.5 Six-month
mortality, stratified by glomerular
filtration rate (GFR) and
biomarker levels. (a) Stratification
by high-sensitivity C-reactive
protein (hs-CRP) levels. (b)
Stratification by Troponin I (cTnl)
levels. (c) Stratification by B-type
natriuretic peptide (BNP) levels.
(From Gibson et al.[24])

The authors concluded that estimation of GFR should be part of the evaluation of any patient presenting with an ACS.

Recently, early coronary angiography and revascularization has been shown to be a more effective strategy for high-risk patients with NSTE-ACS, and current practice guidelines recommend an early invasive strategy in most cases.[25] Therefore, a major issue in CKD patients is the question as to whether renal insufficiency or the coronary revascularization procedure (PCI or CABG) may be the cause of their worsened hospital outcome. In most of the studies focusing on the prognostic role of renal insufficiency in NSTE-ACS, patients were more likely to be treated conservatively with anti-ischemic and antithrombotic agents, while PCI was performed only in patients with recurrent myocardial ischemia. Furthermore, in the studies in which the advantage of an early invasive strategy was demonstrated,[26–28] patients with advanced renal insufficiency, as well as those with an increased risk of bleeding, were excluded. With these limitations, a retrospective study examined the interaction between CrCl, outcomes, and the use of an early invasive strategy in 2190 patients with NSTE-ACS enrolled in the TACTICS-TIMI 18 trial.[17] Irrespective of treatment strategy, mild to moderate decrease in renal function was a potent risk factor for adverse outcome, with a concomitant increase in endpoints such as death, AMI, and rehospitalization at 30 and 180 days. Routine invasive management, however, was associated with a statistically significant reduction in the same endpoints, across most categories of renal insufficiency, at the predictable price of a significant increase in major and minor bleeding. Mueller et al[29] investigated the association between baseline renal function and mortality, after NSTE-ACS, in a cohort of 1400 consecutive, unselected patients treated uniformly very early (within 24 hours of admission, with a median time interval of 5 hours) and predominantly with PCI. Patients with ESRD on dialysis, and with high bleeding risk, were also included in the study. A significantly higher in-hospital and long-term mortality rate was found among patients with a GFR < 60 ml/min per $1.73\,m^2$ of body surface area than among patients with higher GFR. Interestingly, renal function was predictive of long-term mortality, irrespective of the revascularization method applied. Patients with a GFR < 60 ml/min per $1.73\,m^2$ had a hazard ratio of 3.6 (95% CI 1.7–7.6; $P=0.001$), if receiving PCI, and a hazard ratio of 3.9 (95% CI 1.9–8.1; $P<0.001$) if receiving CABG. The hazard ratio was 2.9 (95% CI 0.9–8.8; $P=0.065$) for those being managed with medical treatment only. Thus, this study confirmed that baseline renal function was a strong independent predictor of in-hospital and long-term mortality, and extended this important finding to NSTE-ACS patients treated very early with PCI. It is noteworthy, however, that the cumulative 3-year survival rate of 76.8%, observed among patients with a GFR < 60 ml/min per $1.73\,m^2$, compared favorably with historic controls treated primarily with medical therapy.[5,7,12]

The growing use of PCI in the treatment of NSTE-ACS patients should draw attention to the important impact that CIN may have on the outcome of this population, particularly in the presence of renal dysfunction. In most studies in which the clinical and prognostic impact of CIN after PCI was investigated, patients with NSTE-ACS were included, representing up to 50% of the study population. However, they were never evaluated separately from those undergoing elective PCI because of stable angina.[30–32] Thus, despite a lack of information regarding the precise incidence of CIN in this setting, it seems reasonable to expect that NSTE-ACS patients have an intermediate risk of this complication, which is lower than that presented by patients with STEMI undergoing primary PCI. Indeed, in contrast to primary PCI in which there is no possibility of applying preventive measures such as adequate hydration, CIN prophylaxis is generally feasible in NSTE-ACS patients, and hemodynamic stability is usually obtained before PCI.

Management of acute coronary syndromes in patients with chronic kidney disease

ST-segment elevation myocardial infarction

Treatment of STEMI in patients with CKD is particularly problematic. Traditionally, patients with advanced renal insufficiency and ESRD receiving dialysis have not been included in randomized STEMI trials evaluating either medical or interventional therapies. Thus, only scarce data deriving from limited observational studies are available and, to date, no optimal treatment strategy has been defined for this subgroup of patients. This critical deficiency has been addressed by Berger et al,[33] who compared the patterns of care and the effect of standard AMI therapy on 30-day mortality between 1025 ESRD patients on chronic dialysis (either peritoneal dialysis or hemodialysis) and 145 740 non-ESRD patients. They confirmed that aspirin, beta-blockers, and ACE-inhibitors were less likely to be used in patients on dialysis, even among those considered 'ideal candidates' for these medications, than in patients not receiving dialysis (Figure 5.6). Nevertheless, the authors observed

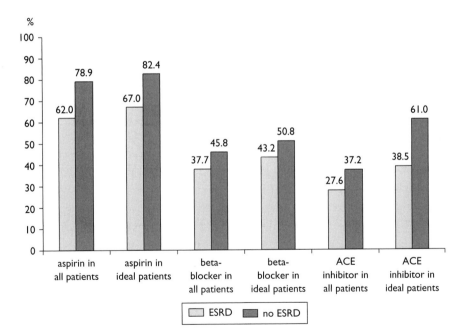

Figure 5.6 *Aspirin, beta-blockers, and angiotensin-converting enzyme (ACE) inhibitors are less likely to be provided to patients with endstage renal disease (ESRD) than to those without ESRD. In an analysis of patients considered ideal for the individual therapies, the overall administration rates were higher, but patients with ESRD still remained less likely to receive the therapy than those without ESRD. The P value for each comparison between ESRD and non-ESRD patients was < 0.001. (From Berger et al.[33])*

a similar absolute reduction in short-term mortality with aspirin, beta-blocker, and ACE inhibitor therapy when comparing the dialysis and non-dialysis groups. Aspirin was associated with a 20.7% absolute reduction in mortality in dialysis patients, and a 22.8% reduction in non-dialysis patients. Beta-blocker therapy was associated with a 13.6% absolute reduction in mortality in both the dialysis and non-dialysis patients. The ACE inhibitor use was associated with a 16.1% absolute reduction in 30-day mortality in dialysis patients and a 5.4% reduction in non-dialysis patients. The reasons for this 'therapeutic nihilism' in dialysis patients and in patients with advanced renal insufficiency suffering from a STEMI are not clear. Concern about further impairment of renal function and toxic side-effects due to reduced drug clearance are potential explanations. Furthermore, patients with renal insufficiency have more comorbidity and, as a consequence, more contraindications to these medications.

Patients with renal insufficiency represent a vulnerable population at higher morbidity and mortality risk; standard medications for secondary prevention (aspirin, beta-blockers, ACE inhibitors and statins) are justified and their use should be encouraged. However, doubts still exist on how they should be treated in the early phase of STEMI. In particular, there are concerns about the use of aggressive reperfusion strategy (fibrinolytic therapy and primary PCI). Undoubtedly, landmark megatrials, such as the Gruppo Italiano per lo Studio della Streptochinasi nell'Infarto Miocardico (GISSI), the International Study of Infarct Survival (ISIS), and the Global Utilization of Streptokinase and Tissue Plasminogen for Occluded Coronary Arteries (GUSTO) trials, have shown the benefit of thrombolytic agents in reducing mortality in patients with STEMI.[34–36] However, in all these trials, no subgroup analysis was performed in patients with renal failure, and scarce data have been published on the use of thrombolytics in CKD patients.

In the study by Wright et al,[9] 13% of the total population received intravenous fibrinolytic therapy and 10% received PCI as a primary treatment. Reperfusion therapy was used less frequently in patients with any degree of renal insufficiency, than in patients without renal insufficiency. However, it was associated with improved long-term survival, but not with reduced risk for in-hospital death. It is conceivable that the potential benefit deriving from early reperfusion could be offset by a morbidity increase, particularly in terms of more bleeding complications after thrombolysis and a higher rate of CIN after primary PCI. Renal insufficiency should not preclude the success rate of percutaneous or pharmacologic reperfusion therapies, but it may be associated with increased incidence of major events.

To evaluate the effects of an invasive management with additional early revascularization, the outcome of 352 patients with STEMI, 24.7% with mild-to-moderate renal insufficiency (sCr ranging from 1.2 to 2.8 mg/dl) was analyzed in a single-center retrospective study.[37] All patients received aspirin, a thrombin inhibitor, and thrombolytic therapy, while early PCI or CABG was performed in 46.8% and 27.6% of patients with normal renal function and 32.2% and 29.9% of those with renal dysfunction. Despite the optimal guideline-based therapy, including invasive management, patients with renal insufficiency showed a significantly higher 30-day and 6-month mortality rate than those with normal renal function (16.1% and 19.5% vs 3.4% and 4.5%, respectively; $P < 0.001$). It is noteworthy, however, that the 30-day and 6-month mortalities were reduced from 22% to 3.6% ($P < 0.03$) and from 25.4% to 7.1% ($P < 0.05$) among renal dysfunction patients who underwent PCI during hospitalization. Thus, this study confirms that mild-to-moderate renal insufficiency in the setting of STEMI is associated with increased mortality,

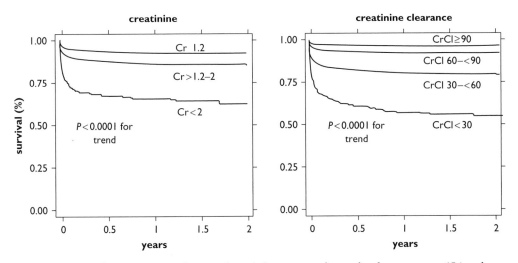

Figure 5.7 *Kaplan–Meier survival curves through 2 years according to baseline creatinine (Cr) and creatinine clearance (CrCl). (From Gibson et al.[38])*

despite extensive use of optimal AMI therapy, but it also suggests that early PCI may be beneficial among such patients.

The influence of renal insufficiency in patients with STEMI receiving fibrinolytic therapy was investigated by Gibson et al,[38] who analyzed pooled data from 16 710 patients enrolled in four studies (TIMI-10A, -10B, and -14, and the inTIME-2 trial). Again, despite appropriate treatment with thrombolytics and adjunctive therapies for AMI (including early PCI in many patients), and even though the epicardial and myocardial reperfusion rates were equivalent, there was a stepwise decrease in survival, going from normal to mildly and severely impaired renal function, that continued through up to 2 years of follow-up (Figure 5.7). The incidence of intracranial hemorrhage was also increased in patients with reduced renal function, suggesting that primary PCI may represent a favorable alternative therapy. Nevertheless, the outcomes of primary PCI in patients with STEMI and renal insufficiency have not been well characterized, because such patients are typically excluded from clinical trials.[39,40]

Sadeghi et al[41] evaluated the potential impact of renal insufficiency in patients undergoing primary PCI and enrolled in the Controlled Abcximab and Device Investigation to Lower Late Angioplasty Complications (CADILLAC) trial. The values of sCr were obtained in 93% of the 1933 patients at hospital admission, and clinical outcomes were assessed as a function of renal insufficiency by examining CrCl strata. At least moderate renal insufficiency, based on a CrCl cut-off of ≤ 60 ml/min, was present in 18% of patients ($n = 350$) who showed a marked increase in the 30-day and 1-year mortality. They had a >9-fold increase in mortality at 30 days, and a 5-fold increase in mortality at one year. Interestingly, this study was the first to report the prognostic relevance of CIN in STEMI patients undergoing primary PCI. Indeed, these patients represent a population at higher risk for CIN than those undergoing elective PCI. Several conditions may contribute to renal injury in this setting. Among them, hypotension or even shock, a large volume of contrast medium, and the impossibility of starting a renal prophylactic therapy are the factors most likely involved. In the CADILLAC trial, CIN, defined as an absolute sCr increase by > 0.5 mg/dl, developed in 4.6% of patients, being three times more prevalent in patients with renal impairment, and was associated with a strikingly worse prognosis (30-day mortality of 16.2% and 1-year mortality of 23.3%). However, the incidence of CIN in this trial was probably underestimated due to the exclusion of patients with known severe renal insufficiency (sCr > 2.0 mg/dl) and to the lack of routine daily sCr measurements. Indeed, sCr levels were assessed at admission, 24 hours after PCI, and at discharge. Therefore, a transient increase in sCr that typically occurs 48 to 72 hours after contrast exposure may have been missed in most patients. The prognostic significance of sCr in STEMI patients treated with primary PCI was also confirmed by a retrospective analysis of 1451 patients drawn from the Heart Institute of Japan Acute Myocardial Infarction (HIJAMI) registry, in which a graded increase of in-hospital death rate (from 3.9% to 17.1% and 34.5%, respectively) was found in the three groups of patients with normal renal function (sCr < 1.2 mg/dl), mild insufficiency (sCr > 1.2 but ≤ 2.0 mg/dl) and severe insufficiency (sCr > 2.0 mg/dl).[42]

The impact of CIN after primary PCI has been investigated in depth in a recent study carried out in our institute.[43] In 208 STEMI patients undergoing primary PCI, the incidence, the clinical predictors, and the clinical consequences of CIN, defined as an absolute increase in sCr > 0.5 mg/dl after PCI, were evaluated. Forty (19%) patients developed CIN. The incidence of this complication was 17% when patients with base-line increased sCr (> 1.5 mg/dl, $n = 11$) were excluded. When CrCl was estimated, 48 (23%) of the 208 patients had a moderately impaired renal function (CrCl < 60 ml/min). Of them, 19 (40%) developed CIN. In contrast, of the 160 patients with a base-line CrCl value ≥ 60 ml/min, only 21 (13%) developed CIN after primary PCI ($P < 0.0001$). Patients with CIN experienced a more complicated in-hospital clinical course (Table 5.1), and their average length of hospital stay was approximately 1.5 times longer than that of patients without CIN (13 ± 7 vs 8 ± 3 days; $P < 0.001$). The overall in-hospital mortality in the entire population was 6.2% ($n = 13$). However, the mortality rate was significantly higher in patients developing CIN than in those without CIN (31% vs 0.6%; $P < 0.0001$). In multivariate analysis, the following variables remained significant independent correlates of CIN: age ≥ 75 years (OR 5.28, 95% CI 1.98–14.05; $P = 0.0009$), anterior STEMI (OR 2.17, 95% CI 0.88–5.34; $P = 0.09$), time-to-reperfusion ≥ 6 hours (OR 2.51, 95% CI 1.01–6.16; $P = 0.04$), contrast agent volume ≥ 300 ml (OR 2.80, 95% CI 1.17–6.68; $P = 0.02$), and the use of an intra-aortic balloon pump (OR 15.51, 95% CI 4.65–51.64; $P < 0.0001$). Using these variables as risk indicators for CIN, a risk scoring system was proposed in which, for each patient, the sum of the number of independent variables (range 0–5) was considered. The incidence of CIN (Figure 5.8), as well as in-hospital mortality (Figure 5.9), revealed a significant gradation as the risk score increased in the study population. Therefore, this study demonstrated that CIN is a frequent complication after primary PCI, even in patients without renal insufficiency, and is associated with increased in-hospital morbidity, mortality, and prolonged hospitalization. In consideration of the widespread application of primary PCI as a reperfusion strategy, innovative preventive approaches aimed at protecting the kidneys from contrast toxicity and ischemic burden during the acute phase of STEMI need to be developed and tested, particularly in high-risk patients, in order to further reduce cardiovascular morbidity and mortality.

Table 5.1   In-hospital clinical complications of patients who developed CIN following primary percutaneous intervention

	CIN (n = 40)	No CIN (n = 168)	P value
CPR, VT, or VF	3 (8%)	7 (4%)	0.41*
High-rate atrial fibrillation	6 (15%)	6 (4%)	0.01*
High-degree conduction disturbances requiring permanent pacemaker	2 (5%)	0 (0%)	0.04*
Acute pulmonary edema	5 (13%)	3 (2%)	0.008*
Respiratory failure requiring mechanical ventilation	8 (20%)	2 (1%)	<0.0001*
Cardiogenic shock requiring intra-aortic balloon counterpulsation	13 (33%)	7 (4%)	<0.0001*
Major bleeding requiring blood transfusion	4 (10%)	5 (3%)	0.07*
Acute renal failure requiring renal replacement therapy	6 (15%)	0 (0%)	<0.0001*
Patients with two or more clinical complications	14 (35%)	4 (3%)	<0.0001*

CIN: contrast-induced nephropathy, CPR: cardiopulmonary resuscitation, VF: ventricular fibrillation; VT: ventricular tachycardia. (From Marenzi et al.[43]).

*By Fisher exact test.

Non-ST-segment elevation acute coronary syndromes

Management of NSTE-ACS patients with renal insufficiency is challenging, due to the increased risk of bleeding and thrombotic events. Data from several clinical trials indicate that new antithrombotic agents and early invasive strategy are of clinical benefit in NSTE-ACS, particularly in high-risk patients. The significant increased mortality of CKD patients suffering from an NSTE-ACS clearly indicates that renal dysfunction represents a strong independent predictor of mortality. Nonetheless, there is still a clear lack of data regarding the optimal management of this complex population, due to the fact that, in most of the NSTE-ACS clinical trials, patients with renal insufficiency were not analyzed separately, or no mention was made of their inclusion or exclusion. Thus, refinement of the antithrombotic strategies among CKD patients in this clinical setting is still a major and unmet need. The challenge is daunting because, on the one hand, renal insufficiency is associated with prolongation of bleeding time and abnormal platelet aggregation

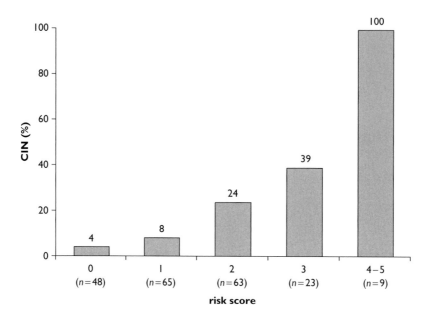

Figure 5.8 *Incidence of contrast-induced nephropathy (CIN) after primary angioplasty according to the risk score; P <0.0001. (From Marenzi et al.[43])*

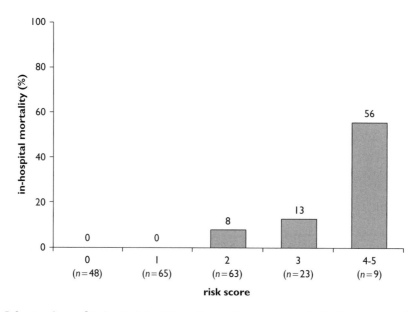

Figure 5.9 *Incidence of in-hospital death in patients with acute myocardial infarction treated with primary angioplasty according to the risk score; P <0.0001. (From Marenzi et al.[43])*

and adhesion,[44] and, on the other hand, a state of hypercoagulation has been demonstrated with high levels of von Willebrand factor,[45] fibrinogen, factors VII, VIII, and XIII, and enhanced thrombin generation.[44] The combination of these alterations puts the patient with CKD at risk, simultaneously, for thrombosis and hemorrhage. Thus, use of well-established antiplatelet drugs, such as aspirin and clopidogrel, should be weighed against bleeding risk in renal patients. Based on the benefit demonstrated in NSTE-ACS, it seems advisable to keep CKD patients on aspirin therapy, with a suggestion for low doses. In addition to aspirin, heparin has become the standard of care in patients with ACS. The two preparations generally available are unfractionated heparin (UFH) and low-molecular-weight heparin (LMWH). A major difference between these two therapeutic agents is their mechanism of clearance: at low doses, UHF is cleared primarily by macrophages and endothelial cell binding, whereas LMWH is cleared primarily by renal mechanisms.[46] Clinical studies on enoxaparin, the most widely used LMWH in NSTE-ACS, excluded patients with renal insufficiency, so that the optimal dosing for renal patients has not been established. A retrospective review showed a significant increase in bleeding events and death in patients with renal insufficiency treated with enoxaparin,[47] suggesting that dosage adjustment is needed in these patients to minimize the hemorrhage risk. Reduction in dose to half, or reduction in frequency of administration to only once daily, may be necessary. However, until conclusive results are available regarding optimal dosing, it may be safer to use UFH in CKD patients presenting with NSTE-ACS. Thus, the pharmacokinetics of aspirin and UHF, although not specifically studied in patients with renal insufficiency, suggest that they are also safe in this population.

Use of newer antithrombotic agents, such as platelet glycoprotein (GP) IIb/IIIa receptor inhibitors, has become the standard of care for the higher-risk NSTE-ACS patients, mainly for those undergoing PCI. However, patients with renal insufficiency were also excluded from entry into most randomized trials investigating GPIIb/IIIa antagonists. Thus, it is not clear whether they may derive the same therapeutic benefit with equivalent safety from these pharmacologic agents as do patients with normal renal function. This question is not surprising, given that renal insufficiency is associated with numerous and well-recognized qualitative platelet abnormalities and coagulation disorders.[48] Moreover, because agents such as tirofiban and eptifibatide are largely cleared through the kidneys, moderate-to-severe renal insufficiency would be expected to increase the mean plasma concentration of these drugs, producing a greater inhibition of platelet aggregation. Since platelet-bound abcximab is eliminated by the reticuloendothelial system,[49] its use in patients with renal insufficiency should not be associated with greater impairment of platelet function. Thus, unlike tirofiban and eptifibatide, abciximab does not require dosing adjustment in CKD patients. Although all major randomized GPIIb/IIIa trials excluded CKD patients, particularly those with severe renal insufficiency, some data about the impact of these agents in this special population may be derived from retrospective trial analysis. It is noteworthy that data extrapolated from the GUSTO-IV ACS study indicate that, in patients with an sCr over 2 mg/dl, abcximab bolus with infusion was associated with a reduction of the combined endpoints of death or myocardial infarction when compared to placebo (15.1% vs 26.8%).[50]

In a recent retrospective subanalysis of the Second Randomized Evaluation in PCI Linking Bivalirudin to Reduced Clinical Events trial (REPLACE-2),[51] within the total randomized population of 5710 patients undergoing PCI (43% of whom because of NSTE-ACS), 886 patients with moderate or severe renal insufficiency showed, as expected, an increased burden of early and late morbidity and mortality. However, bivalirudin (a direct thrombin inhibitor) use among those with renal impairment proved non-inferiority when compared to heparin and GPIIb/IIIa inhibition, with respect to ischemic events.[52] In addition, in the overall population, as well as in patients who had a CrCl < 60 ml/min, bivalirudin was associated with fewer bleeding events. These results are in line with a previous meta-analysis of trials of bivalirudin administration in patients undergoing PCI that showed a reduction of bleeding and ischemic events, with a greater absolute benefit among patients with renal failure.[52] In consideration of the important clinical implications of antithrombotic therapy in this clinical setting, additional randomized trials are warranted to further evaluate the effect of bivalirudin, in terms of ischemic and bleeding complications prevention, in NSTE-ACS patients with renal insufficiency.

Conclusions

Chronic renal insufficiency – of any degree – is present in a substantial proportion of patients with ACS, and represents a potent and independent risk factor for adverse outcome. Although the mechanisms underlying the poor prognosis of this vulnerable population are not fully understood, it is conceivable that the interplay between extensive comorbidities, paradoxical patterns of less aggressive treatment, excess toxicity from conventional therapies, and unique pathobiology of CKD has a considerable role. Unfortunately, data are still limited regarding the value of most therapeutic interventions, because CKD patients with ACS have typically been excluded from randomized trials. Thus, our current challenge is to further study these high-risk patients in prospective randomized trials in order to identify adjunctive pharmacologic therapies and newer interventional strategies that may favorably affect their otherwise poor prognosis. Nevertheless, as long as evidence-based data are not provided to guide clinical practice, all attempts must be made to promote the use of more aggressive therapies, when they can be applied with an acceptable level of safety.

References

1. Go AS, Chertow GM, Fan D, McCulloch CE, Hsu C. Chronic kidney disease and the risk of death, cardiovascular events, and hospitalization. *N Engl J Med* 2004; **351**:1296–305.
2. Gupta R, Birnbaum Y, Uretsky BF. The renal patient with coronary artery disease. Current concepts and dilemmas. *J Am Coll Cardiol* 2004; **44**:1343–53.
3. Masoudi FA, Plomondon ME, Magid DJ, Sales A, Rumsfeld JS. Renal insufficiency and mortality from acute coronary syndromes. *Am Heart J* 2004; **147**:623–9.
4. French JW, Wright RS. Renal insufficiency and worsened prognosis with STEMI. A call for action. *J Am Coll Cardiol* 2003; **42**:1544–6.
5. Herzog CA, Ma JZ, Collins AJ. Poor-long-term survival after acute myocardial infarction among patients on long-term dialysis. *N Engl J Med* 1998; **339**:799–805.
6. Chertow GM, Normand ST, Silva LR, McNeil BJ. Survival after acute myocardial infarction in patients with end-stage renal disease: results from the cooperative cardiovascular project. *Am J Kidney Dis* 2000; **36**:1044–51.
7. Beattie JN, Soman SS, Sandber KR et al. Determinants of mortality after myocardial infarction in patients with advanced renal dysfunction. *Am J Kidney Dis* 2001; **37**:1191–200.

8. McCullough PA, Soman SS, Shah SS et al. Risks associated with renal dysfunction in patients in the coronary care unit. *J Am Coll Cardiol* 2000; **36**:679–84.

9. Wright RS, Reeder GS, Herzog CA et al. Acute myocardial infarction and renal dysfunction: a high-risk combination. *Ann Intern Med* 2002; **137**:563–70.

10. Cockcroft DW, Gault MH. Prediction of creatinine clearance from serum creatinine. *Nephron* 1976; **16**:31–41.

11. Shlipak MG, Heidenreich PA, Noguchi H et al. Association of renal insufficiency with treatment and outcomes after myocardial infarction in elderly patients. *Ann Intern Med* 2002; **137**:555–62.

12. Sorensen CR, Brendorp B, Rask-Madsen C et al. The prognostic importance of creatinine clearance after acute myocardial infarction. *Eur Heart J* 2002; **23**:948–52.

13. Frances CD, Naguchi H, Massie BM et al. Are we inhibited? Renal insufficiency should not preclude the use of ACE inhibition for patients with myocardial infarction and depressed left ventricular function. *Arch Intern Med* 2000; **160**:2645–50.

14. Shlipak MG, Browner WS, Noguchi H et al. Comparison of the effects of angiotensin-converting enzyme inhibitors for patients with myocardial infarction and depressed left ventricular function after myocardial infarction. *Am J Med* 2001; **110**:425–33.

15. Anavekar NS, McMurray JJV, Velazquez EJ et al. Relation between renal dysfunction and cardiovascular outcomes after myocardial infarction. *N Engl J Med* 2004; **351**:1285–95.

16. Santopinto JJ, Fox KAA, Goldber RJ et al. Creatinine clearance and adverse hospital outcomes in patients with acute coronary syndromes: findings from the global registry of acute coronary events (GRACE). *Heart* 2003; **89**:1003–8.

17. Januzzi JL, Cannon CP, DiBaptiste et al for the TACTICS-TIMI 18 Investigators. Effects of renal insufficiency on early invasive management in patients with acute coronary syndromes (the TACTICS-TIMI 18 trial). *Am J Cardiol* 2002; **90**:1246–9.

18. James SK, Lindahl B, Siegbahn A et al. N-terminal pro-brain natriuretic peptide and other risk markers for the separate prediction of mortality and subsequent myocardial infarction in patients with unstable coronary artery disease: a Global Utilization of Strategies to Open occluded arteries (GUSTO)-IV substudy. *Circulation* 2003; **108**:275–81.

19. Masoudi FA, Plomondon ME, Magid DJ, Sales A, Rumsfeld JS. Renal insufficiency and mortality from acute coronary syndromes. *Am Heart J* 2004; **147**:623–9.

20. Wilson S, Foo K, Cunningham J et al. Renal function and risk stratification in acute coronary syndromes. *Am J Cardiol* 2003; **91**:1051–4.

21. Naidu SS, Seltzer F, Jacobs A et al. Renal insufficiency is an independent predictor of mortality after percutaneous coronary intervention. *Am J Cardiol* 2003; **92**:1160–4.

22. Keeley EC, Kadakia R, Soman S, Borzak S, McCullough PA. Analysis of long-term survival after revascularization in patients with chronic kidney disease presenting with acute coronary syndromes. *Am J Cardiol* 2003; **92**:509–14.

23. Gurm HS, Lincoff AM, Kleiman NS et al. Double jeopardy of renal insufficiency and anemia in patients undergoing percutaneous coronary interventions. *Am J Cardiol* 2004; **94**:30–4.

24. Gibson CM, Dumaine RL, Gelfand EV et al. Association of glomerular filtration rate on presentation with subsequent mortality in non-ST-segment elevation acute coronary syndrome; observations in 13307 patients in five TIMI trials. *Eur Heart J* 2004; **25**:1998–2005.

25. Bertrand ME, Simoons ML, Fox KA et al. Management of acute coronary syndromes in patients presentin without persistent ST-segment elevation. *Eur Heart J* 2002; **23**:1809–40.

26. Wallentin L, Lagerqvist B, Husted S et al. Outcome at 1 year after an invasive compared with a non-invasive strategy in unstable coronary artery disease: the FRISC II invasive randomized trial. FRISC II Investigators. Fast Revascularization during Instability in Coronary artery disease. *Lancet* 2000; **356**:9–16.

27. Cannon CP, Weintraub WS, Demopoulos LA et al. TACTICS (Treat Angina with Aggrastat and Determine Cost of Therapy with an Invasive or Conservative Strategy). Thrombolysis in Myocardial Infarction 18 Investigators. *N Engl J Med* 2001; **344**:1879–87.

28. Fox KAA, Poole-Wilson PA, Henderson RA et al. Interventional versus conservative treatment for patients with unstable angina or non-ST-elevation myocardial infarction: the British Heart Foundation RITA 3 randomized trial. *Lancet* 2002; **360**:743–51.

29. Mueller C, Neumann FJ, Perruchoud AP, Buettner HJ. Renal function and long term mortality after unstable angina/non-ST segment elevation myocardial infarction treated very early and predominantly with percutaneous coronary intervention. *Heart* 2004; **90**:902–7.

30. Bartholomew BA, Harjai KJ, Dukkipati S et al. Impact of nephropathy after percutaneous coronary intervention and a method for risk stratification. *Am J Cardiol* 2004; **93**:1515–19.

31. Gruberg L, Mintz GS, Mehran R et al. The prognostic implications of further renal function deterioration within 48 h of interventional coronary procedures in patients with pre-existent chronic renal insufficiency. *J Am Coll Cardiol* 2000; **36**:1542–8.

32. Mehran R, Aymong ED, Nikolsky E et al. A simple risk score for prediction of contrast-induced nephropathy after percutaneous coronary intervention. *J Am Coll Cardiol* 2004; **44**:1393–9.

33. Berger AK, Duval S, Krumholz HK. Aspirin, beta-blocker, and angiotensin-converting enzyme inhibitor therapy in patients with end-stage renal disease and an acute myocardial infarction. *J Am Coll Cardiol* 2003; **42**:201–8.

34. Gruppo Italiano per lo Studio della Streptochinasi nell'Infarto Miocardico (GISSI). Effectiveness of intravenous thrombolytic treatment in acute myocardial infarction. *Lancet* 1986; **1**:397–402.

35. ISIS-2 (Second International Study of Infarct Survival) Collaborative Group. Randomised trial of intravenous streptokinase, oral aspirin, both, or neither among 17,187 cases of suspected acute myocardial infarction: ISIS-2. *Lancet* 1988; **2**:349–60.

36. The GUSTO investigators. An international randomized trial comparing four thrombolytic strategies for acute myocardial infarction. *N Engl J Med* 1993; **329**:673–82.

37. Hobbach HP, Gibson CM, Giugliano RP et al. The prognostic value of serum creatinine on admission in fibrinolytic-eligible patients with acute myocardial infarction. *J Thromb Thrombol* 2003; **16**:167–74.

38. Gibson CM, Pinto DS, Murphy SA et al. Association of creatinine and creatinine clearance on presentation in acute myocardial infarction with subsequent mortality. *J Am Coll Cardiol* 2003; **42**:1535–43.

39. Stone GW, Grines CL, Cox DA et al. Comparison of angioplasty with stenting, with or without abcximab, in acute myocardial infarction. *N Engl J Med* 2002; **346**:957–66.

40. Grines CL, Cox DA, Stone GW. Coronary angioplasty with or without stent implantation for acute myocardial infarction. Stent Primary Angioplasty in Myocardial Infarction Study Group. *N Engl J Med* 1999; **341**:1949–56.

41. Sadeghi HM, Stone GW, Grines CL et al. Impact of renal insufficiency in patients undergoing primary angioplasty for acute myocardial infarction. *Circulation* 2003; **108**:2769–75.

42. Yamaguchi J, Kasanuki H, Ishii Y et al. Prognostic significance of serum creatinine concentration for in-hospital mortality in patients with acute myocardial infarction who underwent successful primary percutaneous coronary intervention (from the Heart Institute of Japan Acute Myocardial Infarction [HIJAMI] registry). *Am J Cardiol* 2004; **93**:1526–8.

43. Marenzi G, Lauri G, Assanelli E et al. Contrast-induced nephropathy in patients undergoing primary angioplasty for acute myocardial infarction. *J Am Coll Cardiol* 2004; **44**:1780–5.

44. Sagripanti A, Barsotti G. Bleeding and thrombosis in chronic uremia. *Nephron* 1997; **75**:125–39.

45. Stam F, van Guldener C, Schalkwijk CG et al. Impaired renal function is associated with markers of endothelial dysfunction and increased inflammatory activity. *Nephrol Dial Transplant* 2003; **18**:892–8.

46. Boneu B, Caranobe C, Cadroy Y et al. Pharmacokinetic studies of standard unfractionated heparin, and low molecular weight heparins in the rabbit. *Semin Thromb Haemost* 1988; **14**:18–27.

47. Fernandez JS, Sadaniantz BT, Sadaniantz A. Review of antithrombotic agents used for acute coronary syndromes in renal patients. *Am J Kidney Dis* 2003; **42**:446–55.

48. Noris M, Remuzzi G. Uremic bleeding: closing the circle after 30 years of controversies? *Blood* 1999; **94**:2569–74.

49. Bhatt DL, Topol EJ. Current role of platelet glycoprotein IIb/IIIa inhibitors in acute coronary syndromes. *JAMA* 2000; **284**:1549–58.

50. Freeman RV, Mehta RH, Al Badr W et al. Influence of concurrent renal dysfunction on outcomes of patients with acute coronary syndromes and implications of the use of glycoprotein IIb/IIIa inhibitors. *J Am Coll Cardiol* 2003; **41**:718–24.

51. Chew DP, Lincoff AM, Gurm H et al. Bivaluridin versus heparin and glycoprotein IIb/IIIa inhibition among patients with renal impairment undergoing percutaneous coronary intervention (a subanalysis of the REPLACE-2 trial). *Am J Cardiol* 2005; **95**:581–5.

52. Chew DP, Bhatt DL, Kimball W et al. Bivalirudin provides increasing benefit with decreasing renal function: a meta-analysis of randomized trials. *Am J Cardiol* 2003; **92**:919–23.

6. RENOVASCULAR DISEASE IN PATIENTS WITH CORONARY ARTERY DISEASE

Michael H Duong, Craig A Thompson, and Aaron V Kaplan

Introduction

Renovascular disease (RVD) is a generalized term referring to lesions of the main renal artery, including stenoses, aneurysms, and occlusions. RVD has emerged as an important comorbidity impacting the care of patients with coronary artery disease (CAD). RVD is the most common cause of secondary hypertension and the second leading cause of renal insufficiency after diabetic nephropathy.[1] An increased awareness coupled with the availability of new diagnostic techniques has led to a rising number of patients identified with RVD. The risk factors and pathophysiology leading to RVD appear to be similar to those for CAD. The vast majority of patients with RVD have renal artery stenosis (RAS), traditionally defined as a critical narrowing in the lumen of the main renal artery,[2] although branch vessel and accessory vessel disease may coexist. Rarely aneurysms of the renal vasculature may also be encountered. Moreover, RVD has been identified as an independent predictor of increased adverse coronary events.[3] The severity of RAS has been shown to correlate with mortality in a long-term population study.[4] In fact current data suggest survival is worse in patients with renovascular hypertension compared to those with essential hypertension.[2,5,6] Because of its prevalence among patients with coronary artery disease in the cardiac catheterization suites and its relationship to hypertension, renal insufficiency, volume overload, and poor outcomes, it is important for the cardiovascular specialist to have a complete understanding of this disease. Furthermore, physicians performing diagnostic and interventional cardiology catheterization procedures need to have a low threshold for performing renal angiography (selective and non-selective) to better identify patients with RAS.

Etiologies and epidemiology

The two most common etiologies of renal artery stenosis are atherosclerosis (90%) and fibromuscular dysplasia (FMD). FMD, first described in 1938 by Leadbetter and Burkland, accounts for less than 10% of RAS cases encountered.[7] Other rarer causes of RVD include vasculitis, neurofibromatosis, congenital bands, pheochromocytoma, extrinsic compression, emboli, aortic dissection, and radiation arteriopathy.[2] FMD is a developmental disorder involving the arterial intima, media, and adventitia. Several histopathologic variants have been identified based on dysplastic involvement of the arterial intima, media, or peri-adventitia. In comparison to atherosclerosis, fibromuscular dysplasia most often affects women, becoming clinically apparent between late adolescence and adulthood (ages 15–50) and usually involves the distal main renal artery or the intra-renal branches.[8] Its incidence increases among smokers and patients with hypertension. There is also evidence suggesting a familial inheritance pattern.[9] The classic 'string of beads' appearance on angiography is seen most often with medial fibroplasias of the arterial wall and represents alternating sequences of stenoses and aneurysms.

Atherosclerotic renal artery stenosis (ARAS) primarily affects men over the age of 45 and is by far the more likely etiology to coexist with CAD. ARAS is caused by extension of aortic athero-sclerotic plaque into the renal arteries and thus typically leads to aorto-ostial stenosis. The true incidence of renal artery stenosis in the general population is unknown. However, it is estimated to account for 1–5% of all hypertensive patients.[1,10–13] A more recent community-based study suggests nearly 7% of all patients over age 65 have underlying renovascular disorders.[14] This is concordant with the growing number of patients with chronic kidney disease (CKD). By 2010 in the United States alone, it is projected that over 100 000 patients will end up on dialysis due to inadequate identification and treatment of ARAS.[15] RAS has now emerged as the most common potentially reversible disorder leading to renal replacement therapy.[4]

ARAS can occur as an isolated renal lesion, but is much more common in patients with coro-nary atherosclerosis or with atherosclerotic disease in other vascular beds (~10–30% incidence).[16] Among patients who are referred for cardiac catheterization, the incidence of disease ranges from 11 to 24%.[17–21] Moreover Leandri et al observed an incidence of ARAS in 467 cardiac catheteriza-tion patients having multivessel coronary disease and 'mild' renal insufficiency to be nearly 33%.[22] This incidence was increased in the patient subset with multidrug-resistant hypertension (usually defined as resistance to three or more antihypertensive medications at relevant dosages, one being a diuretic), renal insufficiency, and episodic congestive heart failure and flash pulmonary edema not explained by coronary disease or poor systolic function.

Pathophysiology

Much of the current knowledge regarding renovascular pathophysiology stems from the seminal experiments of Harry Goldblatt (1891–1977). In 1934, Dr Goldblatt demonstrated hypertensive responses to renal artery constriction in dog models. The two-kidney, one-clip (2K,1C) model of renal stenosis is thought to be a surrogate for unilateral, renal artery stenosis in patients (Figure 6.1). The decrease in flow and pressure created by this preparation leads to activation of the renin–angiotensin axis starting with the secretion of renin, which cleaves angiotensinogen to angiotensin I (AI). Angiotensin-converting enzyme (ACE) converts AI to angiotensin II (AII), a potent stimulator of increased blood pressure by direct vasoconstriction, aldosterone stimulation, and redistribution of renal blood flow. Salt and water are excreted by the 'normal' or non-stenosed kidney by pressure natriuresis. Hence, the 2K,1C model, or unilateral RAS, leads to a state of renin-dependent hypertension. Although the 2K,1C model has provided important insights into the pathoanatomy and pathophysiology of RVD, it does not model the impact of dis-ease within the 'normal' kidney. The role of long-standing hypertension and diabetes on the 'nor-mal' kidney appears to amplify the disease processes driving RVD.

The one-kidney, one-clip (1K,1C) Goldblatt model provides insights into the clinical situation of global renal ischemia (e.g. bilateral RAS or RAS to a solitary functioning kidney) (Figure 6.2).

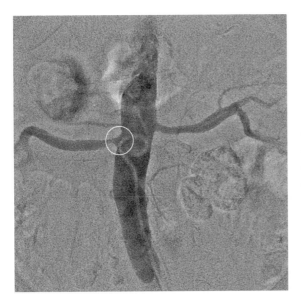

Figure 6.1   *Unilateral stenosis (circle) is demonstrated in the proximal right renal artery. If the contralateral kidney is spared from chronic damage and compromised excretory function, this anatomic scenario would be expected to mimic the Goldblatt 2-kidney, 1-clip (2K,1C) model, resulting in pressure natriuresis from the non-stenosed kidney and a renin-dependent, hypertensive state.*

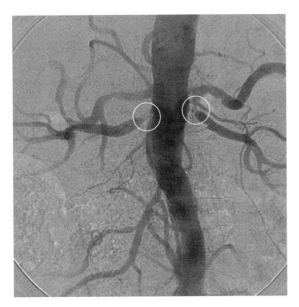

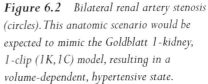

Figure 6.2   *Bilateral renal artery stenosis (circles). This anatomic scenario would be expected to mimic the Goldblatt 1-kidney, 1-clip (1K,1C) model, resulting in a volume-dependent, hypertensive state.*

In this model, a decrease in blood flow and pressure to the kidneys initially stimulates the renin–angiotensin cascade. However, in this circumstance, a 'normal' kidney is not present to secrete sodium and water. Sodium and water are then retained. Intravascular volume is increased and the renin cascade is subsequently suppressed. This scenario thus creates a cycle of volume-dependent hypertension. In the clinical setting of global renovascular ischemia, kidney function may be highly dependent on angiotensin II (and relative efferent arteriolar constriction) to maintain glomerular filtration. This can be a fragile circumstance easily perturbed by ACE inhibitors and other agents, particularly in a sodium-depleted state. When RAS is identified, its impact on renal function may be variable. Overall filtering and excretory capacity may be impaired on the basis of global renal ischemia (1K,1C), isolated renal ischemia (2K,1C) with compromise of contralateral renal function due to underlying comorbidities (e.g. hypertensive nephrosclerosis, diabetic nephropathy, etc.), or related exclusively to primary renal diseases with RAS simply as an incidental finding. The complex pathophysiology of RAS and multifactorial coexistent conditions can often make prediction of response to renal revascularization in the patient care setting difficult.

Clinical presentation

RAS is a complex clinical entity leading to a wide spectrum of clinical manifestations ranging from asymptomatic to combinations of hypertension, renal insufficiency, and volume disturbances (e.g. pulmonary edema/'diastolic dysfunction', peripheral edema, ascites, and/or frank anasarca). Repeated episodes of unexplained heart failure or 'flash' pulmonary edema are emerging as strong indicators for the presence of RVD. Patients with bilateral RAS or stenosis to a solitary functioning kidney, even with preserved left ventricular systolic function, often experience serious sequelae. Clinical suggestions for RAS include: abrupt onset of hypertension (HTN) in patients < 50 years of age, an accelerated rise in blood pressure over usual measurements, HTN with evidence of endorgan damage, multidrug-resistant HTN, unexplained azotemia and cardiac disturbance syndromes (pulmonary edema not adequately explained on the basis of heart disease). Physical exam findings including abdominal/flank bruits and volume overload may be helpful, although the absence of these findings should not be misconstrued as 'ruling out' RVD. Patients with vascular disease in any other distribution should be evaluated for RAS, especially in the presence of these clinical findings. As previously discussed, renal function may deteriorate with administration of ACE inhibitors due to relative loss of efferent arteriolar tone and subsequent decrease in glomerular filtration.

The natural history of RAS is poorly understood due to past inability to identify and follow patients longitudinally with non-invasive techniques. Only recently with advancements in imaging (i.e. renal duplex ultrasonography [RDUS], computer-tomographic angiography [CTA], magnetic resonance angiography [MRA]) have we begun to better comprehend this complex disease process. A clear understanding of RAS will not be possible until long-term data guided by serial assessments with these technologies are available. Nevertheless, it appears RAS is characterized by progressive atherosclerosis often leading to occlusion, with subsequent renal atrophy with concomitant loss of secretory function.[23] Current consensus suggests three primary clinical criteria for revascularization exist in the setting of RAS:[2,24]

- Hypertension: accelerated or refractory to three different medications including a diuretic. HTN that manifests with endorgan damage (e.g. left ventricular hypertrophy, retinopathy, neurologic-lacunar infarct, renal failure), HTN refractory to medical therapy, and HTN in younger patients (< age 35).
- Renal salvage: sudden and unexplained worsening of renal function or impairment due to antihypertensive agents (especially ACE inhibitor (ACEI) or angiotensin receptor blocker (ARB)).

- Left ventricular diastolic dysfunction: recurrent pulmonary edema in the setting of preserved left ventricular systolic function, especially in patients without obstructive coronary anatomy.

The role for renal revascularization for 'asymptomatic' disease and unilateral disease (for renal preservation) is currently ill defined. In addition, revascularization in chronically damaged kidneys with high resistive index (RI) seems less optimal that those with low RI (see below).[25] However, comparative studies have not been performed to determine whether renal revascularization in patients with high RI is superior to medical therapy alone.

Diagnostic modalities and imaging

Intra-arterial digital subtraction angiography (DSA) is considered the current gold standard for diagnosis of renal artery stenosis[2] (Figure 6.3). However, the procedure is invasive and carries a significant albeit small risk of complications including dissection, embolization, and contrast nephropathy. Several non-invasive tests have been employed over the years as diagnostic alternatives. RDUS has emerged as a commonly employed modality providing both anatomic and physiologic assessment. This widely available, inexpensive, and safe procedure provides two-dimensional ultrasound and Doppler flow evaluation of the kidneys and renal arteries. Assessment of renal span and presence of aneurysms, cysts, or hydronephrosis can be obtained. Increased renal arterial velocities (peak systolic velocity > 200 cm/s) or an elevated renal-to-aortic flow velocity ratio (> 3.5) is considered diagnostic for a functional stenosis and correlates with narrowings of 60–99%.[2] Duplex scanning can also be used to assess renal resistive index RI values, defined as $(1 - (\text{end-diastolic velocity [cm/s]}/\text{peak systolic velocity [cm/s]}) \times 100)$. The RI is regarded as an indicator of renal arterial impedance due to microvascular disease/nephrosclerosis.[25] RI values appear to be an important parameter in determining benefit from renal revascularization (which is discussed later in this chapter). Another advantage of RDUS is the ability to assess arterial

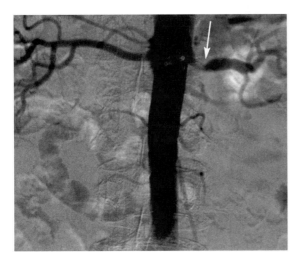

Figure 6.3 *Critical left renal artery stenosis (arrow) on digital subtraction, non-selective renal angiography in a patient with resistant hypertension on multiple medications including a diuretic.*

patency after stenting. The entire renal artery can be imaged despite the presence of metallic endoprostheses. However, RDUS is not without important limitations. The test is highly operator-dependent and typically requires 1 hour to complete. Imaging the renal arteries is often difficult and frequently not successful in as many as 25% of cases, particularly in the obese patient, and can be further obscured by bowel gas. Small accessory and secondary arteries are often not well imaged by ultrasound. RDUS is highly dependent upon sonographer skill as well as physician expertise in interpretation. Up to 20% of RDUS provides no reliable information.[26,27] When high-quality RDUS studies are available, it should be used as the first-line methodology for evaluating patients at high risk for RVD/RAS. At our institution, the RDUS has a sensitivity of 88% and specificity of 92% compared to invasive angiography. Other institutions have reported numbers as high as 98% and 99%, respectively.[13]

CTA and MRA have emerged as alternative strategies in the diagnostic workup of RAS. Both are non-invasive and provide superior imaging quality compared to RDUS or scintigraphy. CTA requires the use of iodinated contrast media and hence carries the risk of contrast nephropathy. The advent of 16-slice, and newer 64-slice CT technology holds the promise of producing higher-resolution images with reduced acquisition time and lower contrast volumes. Gadolinium enhanced three-dimensional MRA can also provide high-quality images while negating the risk of contrast nephropathy. MRA is limited by costs and availability and is not tolerated by all patients. Moreover, stent-associated artifact limits the utility of MRA as a tool to follow patients after endovascular revascularization/stent procedures. Newer technologies are also available using rotational angiography with three-dimensional reconstructive imaging. Our institution is currently investigating this technology in aiding clinical decision-making during coronary and peripheral catheterization procedures (Figures 6.4 and 6.5).

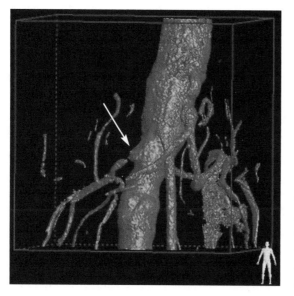

Figure 6.4   *Three-dimensional angiographic reconstruction of a rotational aortogram demonstrating critical right renal artery stenosis on a screening exam of a patient having coronary angiography with a history of difficult-to-control, accelerating hypertension. (Example using Philips Medical System, Dartmouth–Hitchcock Medical Center.)*

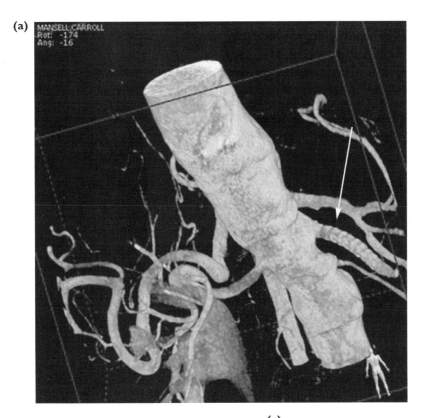

(a)

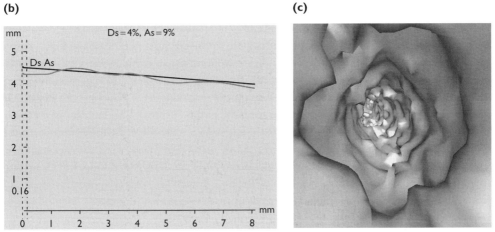

Figure 6.5 *Volume-rendered, three-dimensional reconstruction (3DR, posterior view) after right renal artery stenosis treatment with stent implantation (a, arrow). Rotational angiography with 3DR provides an intraprocedural opportunity to understand special relationships (a), and to perform volumetric assessment for vessel sizing, stenosis measurements, or feedback for procedural success (b) and intravascular 'virtual' angioscopy (c).(Example using Philips Medical System, Dartmouth–Hitchcock Medical Center.)*

Previous studies suggest CTA and MRA have better diagnostic accuracy compared to RDUS and renal scintigraphy, with sensitivities and specificities reaching nearly 100% for both.[10,11,28] More recently, the RADISH study suggested that CTA and MRA are not reproducible or sensitive enough to rule out RAS in hypertensive patients. Both imaging modalities detected only 64% and 62%, respectively, of patients who had DSA findings of renal artery stenosis.[29] These results may have been confounded by an unusually high incidence of FMD (38%) as well as the use of a 50% stenosis as threshold for 'significant' disease. As a result, the sensitivities of both CTA and MRA may have been underestimated.

Captopril renal scintigraphy in recent years has become less popular, particularly with advancements in CTA and MRA. Compared to RDUS, renal scintigraphy is expensive, labor-intensive, and requires the use of radioisotopes. Although previously shown to have sensitivity and specificity exceeding 90%, the test does not provide anatomic information about the renal arteries, and will often demonstrate false-negative results in the high-risk patients with bilateral RAS.[30] Furthermore, renal scintigraphy is less accurate in patients with renal insufficiency, a single functioning kidney, and obstructive uropathy.[1]

Plasma renin level measurements were previously used as a screening test in conjunction with captopril. The test is cumbersome and hindered by both false-negative and false-positive results. As many as 20% of patients with renovascular hypertension will have normal levels.[31,32] Its utility is further limited by the need to discontinue antihypertensive medications that affect renin levels (beta-blockers, ACEI, diuretics). As such, renin measurements now are rarely used.[11]

Treatment

Medical therapy for RAS focuses on aggressive blood pressure control, volume management, and risk factor modification. Management of hypertension in the presence of renovascular disease typically requires combination therapy. The most recent report of the Joint National Committee on prevention, detection, evaluation and treatment of high blood pressure suggests an ACEI or ARB with a thiazide diuretic as part of an antihypertensive regimen in patients with kidney disease.[33] Loop diuretics may also be helpful in cases of volume overload. An increase in creatinine by 30%, hyperkalemia, or severe bilateral RAS may preclude the use of ACEI/ARB as previously discussed. Refractory hypertension, rising creatinine, loss of renal mass, bilateral renal artery disease, volume overload, or an inability to tolerate an ACEI are indications for revascularization. Treatment for traditional atherosclerosis risk factors (i.e. smoking cessation, diabetes, hyperlipidemia) should also be aggressively pursued. Statins have been shown to improve endothelial dysfunction and improve atherosclerotic burden in the coronary tree,[34–37] and early animal studies suggest similar benefits within the renal vasculature.[38] It remains unclear what clinical impact these drugs will have in treating patients with renal artery stenosis.

Renal artery revascularization (RAR)

Revascularization for RAS was traditionally performed via unilateral aorto-renal bypass surgery. Many reconstructive techniques have evolved over the last few decades, including endarterectomy, renal re-implantation, and extra-anatomical bypass surgery. Newer methods for renal artery bypass (e.g. iliorenal, splenorenal, mesenterorenal, and hepatorenal) became more common due to less manipulation required of a concomitantly diseased aorta, with presumed reductions in perioperative complications. Although surgery has the potential to cure or stabilize renal function as well as reverse the progression to endstage renal disease, its morbidity and mortality rates have been relatively high.[39–44] Mortality rates vary depending on operator experience, need for aortic manipulation, and severity of extra-renal vascular disease. Rates vary from 2.1 to 6.1% for extra-anatomical bypass and up to 4.7% for renal endarterectomy.[26,43–45] The best outcomes were observed in younger patients with less disease burden in other vascular territories (particularly coronary, aortic, and cerebrovascular). Advanced renal failure and congestive heart failure also are strong predictors of poorer outcomes with surgical renal revascularization. Because of these risks and the advances in percutaneous techniques, surgery now accounts for only a fraction of all renal revascularization procedures.

Percutaneous transluminal renal angioplasty (PTRA) and stenting

Since Andreas Gruentzig successfully performed the first renal artery angioplasty in 1978,[46] tremendous progress has occurred in the field of percutaneous endovascular renal revascularization. Initial series evaluating angioplasty alone reported a high incidence of recoil (most likely due to aorto-ostial lesion location) with restenosis rates as high as 25%.[47] Stent-supported percutaneous renal intervention has become the revascularization method of choice in most centers (Figure 6.6). Stent scaffolding has improved acute procedural success to ~99% for experienced operators, with similar clinical improvement and durability and very low morbidity and mortality compared to prior

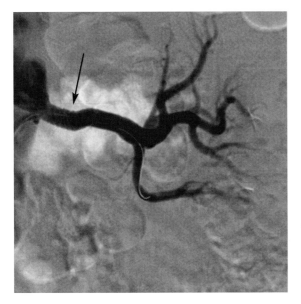

Figure 6.6 *Selective renal angiography post-stenting (arrow) demonstrates no residual stenosis in the patient from Figure 6.3. The hypertension subsequently became well controlled on a reduced number, and dosage, of antihypertensive drugs.*

surgical revascularization experiences.[10,11,26] More recent data demonstrate restenosis rates using bare metal stents as low as 10–14% and a procedural mortality rate ranging from 0.01 to 1%.[48,49]

Efficacy in clinical trials (clinical studies/longitudinal data)

Observational data suggest roughly 10–16% of patients will progress to total arterial occlusion when followed beyond 1–2 years, with increasing probability observed in those arteries with higher-grade obstructions.[11,50,51] In patients with RVD and renal failure, survival without intervention is poor. Mailloux et al reported a median survival of 27 months and 10% survival at 5 years in this population.[52] Other investigators have observed a mortality rate of nearly 40% in patients with bilateral RAS followed for a median of 52 months who did not have renal revascularization.[53,54] To date, no randomized studies designed to evaluate the impact of renal revascularization on 'hard' endpoints such as mortality and/or cardiovascular events have been reported. Most existing studies examine clinical surrogates that impact long-term morbidity and mortality, principally hypertension and renal function. Study design, patient selection, and high crossover rates have limited the usefulness of the available clinical data. Recently, consensus guidelines have been published which may assist in the design and implementation of future clinical trials investigating renal revascularization.[2] This section will focus on the current state of knowledge on the three major trial endpoints: control of hypertension, preservation/improvement in renal function, and reduction of cardiovascular events.

The body of data, albeit small, suggests RAR yields only a modest benefit on blood pressure control. Revascularization, however, rarely cures hypertension (with notable exceptions often seen with FMD). The general expectation is that 60–75% of unselected patients with RAS will have a beneficial response in blood pressure management as a result of renal artery intervention. Small non-randomized series suggest PTRA and renal stenting improve blood pressure control and reduce the number/dosage of drugs.[55] Unfortunately there are only three randomized trials examining percutaneous RAR and its impact on blood pressure control. Two of the studies comprising only 104 patients demonstrated a benefit in hypertension control.[56,57] The largest trial, the Dutch Renal Artery Stenosis Intervention Cooperative study (DRASTIC),[58] randomized 106 patients to either medical therapy or angioplasty alone. At 12 months no difference in hypertension control was reported, although the intervention group required fewer antihypertensive agents. This study was compromised by a high cross-over rate (44%) from medical therapy to angioplasty. Moreover, the use of balloon angioplasty alone makes these data obsolete in the current stent era. In a pooled analysis of these three trials, Nordmann et al demonstrated that intervention was still more effective in reducing blood pressure than medical therapy alone (Figure 6.7). Overall, patients treated with balloon angioplasty were more likely to have patent renal arteries after 12 months, required fewer blood pressure medications, and trended toward having fewer major cardiovascular and renovascular adverse events.[59]

The current body of knowledge regarding the impact of revascularization on renal function is even more difficult to interpret. Prior experience after surgical or percutaneous RAR suggests serum creatinine is stabilized or improved in >70% of patients and deteriorates in the rest.[26,60]

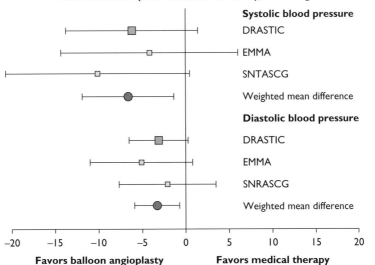

Figure 6.7 *Effect of renal artery angioplasty on blood pressure control in three randomized controlled trials. DRASTIC: Dutch Renal Artery Stenosis Cooperative study; EMMA: Essai Multicentrique Medicaments vs Angioplastie trial; SNRASCG: Scottish and Newcastle Renal Artery Stenosis Collaborative Group trial. (Adapted from Nordmann AJ et al[59]. Permission granted by Excerpta Medica.)*

Watson et al evaluated the effectiveness of renal artery stenting (bilateral RAS or RAS involving a single/solitary functioning kidney) on preserving renal size and function. Stenting was successful in all 61 vessels (33 patients). They observed stabilization of renal function in 72% of patients, and a reduction of function decline in the remainder.[61] In an older review including non-randomized studies ($n = 678$), Leertouwer et al reported improvement in renal function in 30% and stabilization in 38% of patients.[55] Recently Zeller et al reported their 6-year experience in 340 consecutive patients with HTN undergoing stent-supported PTRA.[62] They found a significant decrease in serum creatinine and increase in GFR following intervention. In contrast, none of the three randomized studies cited above were able to demonstrate a major difference in renal function. It is important to reiterate that all these studies were small and not designed to detect improvement in renal function.

The increasing awareness of RAS in patients with severe coronary artery disease and recalcitrant heart failure has led to changes in their management. Numerous small series suggest rapid resolution of pulmonary edema and a decrease in subsequent episodes of congestive heart failure in a majority of patients.[11,63–66] Regrettably, prospective randomized data, like those for renal function, are also lacking. Well-designed, adequately powered, randomized controlled studies are needed to indicate the optimal treatment strategy for RAS patients with congestive heart failure. Until such data are available, we recommend an aggressive percutaneous revascularization strategy in patients with known RAS and recurrent pulmonary edema, especially with preserved systolic function.

There are at least three ongoing randomized studies evaluating the impact of renal artery stenting. Two of the trials (STAR[67] and ASTRAL[68]) are being conducted in Europe and are comparing percutaneous PTRA/stenting with medical therapy. They both designate renal function parameters as primary endpoints. The much anticipated CORAL Trial[69] is a large, prospective, multicenter, randomized trial in the United States comparing cardiovascular and renal events in RAS patients undergoing stent-supported PTRA vs medical therapy alone. Expected enrollment is 1080 patients (during the years 2005–6), with a study duration of 5 years.

Predicting clinical benefit in patients with RAS

RAS is frequently identified angiographically prior to non-invasive physiologic assessment. This has become more common as a result of aggressive screening efforts of patients undergoing cardiac catheterizations and other non-renal peripheral vascular procedures.[18] An emerging dilemma from this practice is the inability to adequately assess lesion significance at the time of angiography and identify those who would most likely benefit from revascularization. Although there is no clear consensus regarding the degree of renal artery narrowing that justifies revascularization, investigators generally define the minimal threshold for an angiographically significant arterial narrowing to be $\geq 50\%$ luminal diameter reduction.[2,70] This is acknowledged as only an approximate guide to the hemodynamic effect of the stenosis. Parameters such as baseline mean blood pressure of > 110 mmHg and bilateral RAS have previously been used to predict improvement in blood pressure after RAR.[60,71] Neither has been prospectively validated. One common in-laboratory procedure is to measure translesional systolic gradients, with a value of > 20 mmHg being considered 'signficant' and an indication for revascularization.[2] This technique has not been standardized nor validated with regard to clinical outcome after revascularization.[70] The best validated procedure that predicts clinical benefit after revascularization is non-invasive Doppler-derived RI, defined as $(1 - (\text{end-diastolic velocity [cm/s]/peak systolic velocity [cm/s]}) \times 100)$. The RI is considered a useful measure of microvascular/nephrosclerosis severity. In a large single-center study, Radermacher et al prospectively evaluated the utility of RI in predicting outcome (HTN control, renal function, mortality) following elective revascularization in RAS patients. Of the 5950 patients screened, 138 underwent renal arterial revascularization (angioplasty or surgery). Patients with RI > 80 ($n = 35$) had a high rate of decrease in renal function (80%) without significant improvement in HTN control. In those with RI < 80 ($n = 96$), 94% had improvement in blood pressure control, with only a small minority (3%) becoming dialysis dependent.[25] The impact of revascularization on patients with high RI values appears to be marginal. Thus, RI remains the only physiologic characteristic that has been clinically validated as a predictor of outcomes.[11,28,70] In an effort to provide a 'real-time' physiologic assessment of RAS identified as part of a catheterization procedure, we are using an invasive technique by which RI values can be readily assessed. All patients identified with RAS in the catheterization lab undergo adjunctive selective renal angiography and assessment of renal flow velocities and RI calculations using a Doppler-tipped guide wire that is placed in the renal arteries. These invasively derived values are then compared to values derived from standard non-invasive RDUS. This protocol is in the process of being validated as part of the ongoing Renal Artery Stenosis Invasive Doppler Trial at our institution.

A number of other non-invasive techniques evaluating the physiologic importance of RAS are currently under investigation, including measurements of parenchymal volume and perfusion by MRA and ultra-fast CTA.[72–74] Positron emission tomography (PET), which measures metabolic activity, has the potential for identifying tissue viability. PET could be a valuable adjunct to distinguish 'hibernating' parenchyma from that which is unrecoverable, as has been demonstrated in studies of myocardial ischemia.[73,75] Fascinating data have recently surfaced suggesting elevated baseline brain natriuretic peptide may also be a good predictor of beneficial blood pressure response after stent revascularization.[76] Further studies will be required to fully validate the use of these technologies as well as to provide an understanding of how they can best be incorporated into routine practice.

Conclusions

Renal artery stenosis frequently co-exists with coronary artery disease. Its complex pathophysiology and its optimal clinical management are incompletely understood. Presentations can vary from quiescent to clinically apparent with malignant hypertension, renal failure, and/or volume disturbance. These phenotypic manifestations can occur alone or in combination, thus creating difficulty in standardizing diagnosis and management strategies. Therefore it is imperative for the cardiovascular specialist to be aware and knowledgeable of RAS. Efforts should be made to systematically screen for RAS when clinical features such as multidrug-resistant hypertension, progressive renal failure, and repeated episodes of pulmonary edema with preserved ventricular systolic function are encountered. Renal duplex ultrasonography, magnetic resonance angiography, and computed tomographic angiography are the best, non-invasive, first-line imaging modalities for diagnosis. The decision for which test is appropriate is best determined by local expertise. For patients who are undergoing cardiac catheterization or other vascular angiography, we recommend performing adjunctive non-selective renal angiography in those with clinical features suggestive of RAS. At minimum, these patients warrant aggressive medical therapy and surveillance for disease progression. Revascularization should be considered in patients with significant renal arterial disease with resistant hypertension, compromised renal function, or volume overload/pulmonary edema. An additional consideration is 'prophylactic' stenting for critical renal stenosis in the sole remaining/functioning kidney. It is important to reiterate that our understanding of renal vascular disease is rapidly changing. As the applications of emerging technologies to assess anatomic and functional features of RAS continue to grow, so will our understanding of this disease process.

References

1. Radermacher J, Haller H. The right diagnostic work-up: investigating renal and renovascular disorders. *J Hypertens Suppl* 2003; **21(Suppl 2)**:S19–24.
2. Rundback JH, Sacks D, Kent KC et al. Guidelines for the reporting of renal artery revascularization in clinical trials. *J Vasc Interv Radiol* 2003; **14**:S477–92.

3. Edwards MS, Craven TE, Burke GL, Dean RH, Hansen KJ. Renovascular disease and the risk of adverse coronary events in the elderly: a prospective, population-based study. *Arch Intern Med* 2005; **165**:207–13.

4. Buller CE, Nogareda JG, Ramanathan K et al. The profile of cardiac patients with renal artery stenosis. *J Am Coll Cardiol* 2004; **43**:1606–13.

5. Johansson M, Herlitz H, Jensen G, Rundqvist B, Friberg P. Increased cardiovascular mortality in hypertensive patients with renal artery stenosis. Relation to sympathetic activation, renal function and treatment regimens. *J Hypertens* 1999; **17**:1743–50.

6. Implications of the systolic hypertension in the elderly program. The Systolic Hypertension in the Elderly Program Cooperative Research Group. *Hypertension* 1993; **21**:335–43.

7. Slovut DP, Olin JW. Fibromuscular dysplasia. *N Engl J Med* 2004; **350**:1862–71.

8. Fernando D, Garasic J. Percutaneous intervention for renovascular disease: rationale and patient selection. *Curr Opin Cardiol* 2004; **19**:582–8.

9. Pannier-Moreau I, Grimbert P, Fiquet-Kempf B et al. Possible familial origin of multifocal renal artery fibromuscular dysplasia. *J Hypertens* 1997; **15**:1797–801.

10. Bokhari SW, Faxon DP. Current advances in the diagnosis and treatment of renal artery stenosis. *Rev Cardiovasc Med* 2004; **5**:204–15.

11. Olin JW. Renal artery disease: diagnosis and management. *Mt Sinai J Med* 2004; **71**:73–85.

12. Ram CV. Renovascular hypertension. *Curr Opin Nephrol Hypertens* 1997; **6**:575–9.

13. Olin JW, Piedmonte MR, Young JR et al. The utility of duplex ultrasound scanning of the renal arteries for diagnosing significant renal artery stenosis. *Ann Intern Med* 1995; **122**:833–8.

14. Hansen KJ, Edwards MS, Craven TE et al. Prevalence of renovascular disease in the elderly: a population-based study. *J Vasc Surg* 2002; **36**:443–51.

15. Fatica RA, Port FK, Young EW. Incidence trends and mortality in end-stage renal disease attributed to renovascular disease in the United States. *Am J Kidney Dis* 2001; **37**:1184–90.

16. Edwards MS, Hansen KJ, Craven TE et al. Associations between renovascular disease and prevalent cardiovascular disease in the elderly: a population-based study. *Vasc Endovascular Surg* 2004; **38**:25–35.

17. Textor SC. Pitfalls in imaging for renal artery stenosis. *Ann Intern Med* 2004; **141**:730–1.

18. White CJ. Screening renal artery angiography at the time of cardiac catheterization. *Catheter Cardiovasc Interven* 2003; **60**:295–6.

19. Khosla S, Kunjummen B, Manda R et al. Prevalence of renal artery stenosis requiring revascularization in patients initially referred for coronary angiography. *Catheter Cardiovasc Interven* 2003; **58**:400–3.

20. Weber-Mzell D, Kotanko P, Schumacher M, Klein W, Skrabal F. Coronary anatomy predicts presence or absence of renal artery stenosis. A prospective study in patients undergoing cardiac catheterization for suspected coronary artery disease. *Eur Heart J* 2002; **23**:1684–91.

21. Harding MB, Smith LR, Himmelstein SI et al. Renal artery stenosis: prevalence and associated risk factors in patients undergoing routine cardiac catheterization. *J Am Soc Nephrol* 1992; **2**:1608–16.

22. Leandri M, Lipiecki J, Lipiecka E et al. Prevalence of renal artery stenosis in patients undergoing cardiac catheterization: when should abdominal aortography be performed? Results in 467 patients. *J Radiol* 2004; **85**:627–33.

23. Zeller T, Muller C, Frank U et al. Survival after stenting of severe atherosclerotic ostial renal artery stenoses. *J Endovasc Ther* 2003; **10**:539–45.

24. Jaff MR. Hypertension and renal artery stenosis: a complex clinical scenario. *J Am Osteopath Assoc* 2000; **100**:S5–9.

25. Radermacher J, Chavan A, Bleck J et al. Use of Doppler ultrasonography to predict the outcome of therapy for renal-artery stenosis. *N Engl J Med* 2001; **344**:410–17.

26. Safian RD, Textor SC. Renal-artery stenosis. *N Engl J Med* 2001; **344**:431–42.

27. Hansen KJ, Tribble RW, Reavis SW. Renal duplex sonography: evaluation of clinical utility. *J Vasc Surg* 1990; **12**:227–36.

28. Olin JW, Kaufman JA, Bluemke DA et al. Atherosclerotic Vascular Disease Conference: Writing Group IV: imaging. *Circulation* 2004; **109**:2626–33.

29. Vasbinder GB, Nelemans PJ, Kessels AG et al. Accuracy of computed tomographic angiography and magnetic resonance angiography for diagnosing renal artery stenosis. *Ann Intern Med* 2004; **141**:674–82; discussion 682.

30. Mann SJ. Captopril renal scans for detecting renal artery stenosis. *Arch Intern Med* 2003; **163**:630; author reply 630–1.

31. Kaplan N, Rose B. Screening for renovascular hypertension. In: Rose B, ed. *UpToDate*. Wellesley, MA; 2004.

32. Wilcox CS. Use of angiotensin-converting-enzyme inhibitors for diagnosing renovascular hypertension. *Kidney Int* 1993; **44**:1379–90.

33. Chobanian AV, Bakris GL, Black HR et al. The Seventh Report of the Joint National Committee on Prevention, Detection, Evaluation, and Treatment of High Blood Pressure: the JNC 7 report. *JAMA* 2003; **289**:2560–72.

34. Nissen SE, Tuzcu EM, Schoenhagen P et al. Effect of intensive compared with moderate lipid-lowering therapy on progression of coronary atherosclerosis: a randomized controlled trial. *JAMA* 2004; **291**:1071–80.

35. Mohler E. Endothelial dysfunction. In: Rose B, ed. *UpToDate*. Wellesley, MA; 2004.

36. Yokoyama I, Momomura S, Ohtake T et al. Improvement of impaired myocardial vasodilatation due to diffuse coronary atherosclerosis in hypercholesterolemics after lipid-lowering therapy. *Circulation* 1999; **100**:117–22.

37. Lefer AM, Campbell B, Shin YK et al. Simvastatin preserves the ischemic-reperfused myocardium in normocholesterolemic rat hearts. *Circulation* 1999; **100**:178–84.

38. Zhu X, Chade A, Ritman E, Lerman A, Lerman LO. Simvastatin preserves renal microvascular structure in renal artery stenosis. *J Am Coll Cardiol* 2005; **45**:378a.

39. Weibull H, Bergqvist D, Bergentz SE et al. Percutaneous transluminal renal angioplasty versus surgical reconstruction of atherosclerotic renal artery stenosis: a prospective randomized study. *J Vasc Surg* 1993; **18**:841–50; discussion 850–2.

40. Dorros G, Jaff M, Mathiak L, He T. Multicenter Palmaz stent renal artery stenosis revascularization registry report: four-year follow-up of 1,058 successful patients. *Catheter Cardiovasc Interven* 2002; **55**:182–8.

41. Cambria RP, Brewster DC, L'Italien GJ et al. Renal artery reconstruction for the preservation of renal function. *J Vasc Surg* 1996; **24**:371–80; discussion 380–2.

42. Hallett JW Jr, Fowl R, O'Brien PC et al. Renovascular operations in patients with chronic renal insufficiency: do the benefits justify the risks? *J Vasc Surg* 1987; **5**:622–7.

43. Hansen KJ, Starr SM, Sands RE et al. Contemporary surgical management of renovascular disease. *J Vasc Surg* 1992; **16**:319–30; discussion 330–1.

44. Novick AC, Ziegelbaum M, Vidt DG et al. Trends in surgical revascularization for renal artery disease. Ten years' experience. *JAMA* 1987; **257**:498–501.

45. Clair DG, Belkin M, Whittemore AD, Mannick JA, Donaldson MC. Safety and efficacy of transaortic renal endarterectomy as an adjunct to aortic surgery. *J Vasc Surg* 1995; **21**:926–33; discussion 934.

46. Gruntzig A, Kuhlmann U, Vetter W et al. Treatment of renovascular hypertension with percutaneous transluminal dilatation of a renal-artery stenosis. *Lancet* 1978; **1**:801–2.

47. Dorros G, Jaff M, Jain A, Dufek C, Mathiak L. Follow-up of primary Palmaz-Schatz stent placement for atherosclerotic renal artery stenosis. *Am J Cardiol* 1995; **75**:1051–5.

48. Cognet F, Garcier JM, Dranssart M et al. Percutaneous transluminal renal angioplasty in atheroma with renal failure: long-term outcomes in 99 patients. *Eur Radiol* 2001; **11**:2524–30.

49. van de Ven PJ, Kaatee R, Beutler JJ et al. Arterial stenting and balloon angioplasty in ostial atherosclerotic renovascular disease: a randomised trial. *Lancet* 1999; **353**:282–6.

50. White CJ. Renal artery revascularization: percutaneous stent placement is the standard of practice. *Vasc Med* 2002; **7**:3–4.

51. Greco BA, Breyer JA. The natural history of renal artery stenosis: who should be evaluated for suspected ischemic nephropathy? *Semin Nephrol* 1996; **16**:2–11.

52. Mailloux LU, Napolitano B, Bellucci AG et al. Renal vascular disease causing end-stage renal disease, incidence, clinical correlates, and outcomes: a 20-year clinical experience. *Am J Kidney Dis* 1994; **24**:622–9.

53. Conlon PJ, Athirakul K, Kovalik E et al. Survival in renal vascular disease. *J Am Soc Nephrol* 1998; **9**:252–6.

54. Conlon PJ, Little MA, Pieper K, Mark DB. Severity of renal vascular disease predicts mortality in patients undergoing coronary angiography. *Kidney Int* 2001; **60**:1490–7.

55. Leertouwer TC, Gussenhoven EJ, Bosch JL et al. Stent placement for renal arterial stenosis: where do we stand? A meta-analysis. *Radiology* 2000; **216**:78–85.

56. Plouin PF, Chatellier G, Darne B, Raynaud A. Blood pressure outcome of angioplasty in atherosclerotic renal artery stenosis: a randomized trial. Essai Multicentrique Medicaments vs Angioplastie (EMMA) Study Group. *Hypertension* 1998; **31**:823–9.

57. Webster J, Marshall F, Abdalla M et al. Randomised comparison of percutaneous angioplasty vs continued medical therapy for hypertensive patients with atheromatous renal artery stenosis. Scottish and Newcastle Renal Artery Stenosis Collaborative Group. *J Hum Hypertens* 1998; **12**:329–35.

58. van Jaarsveld BC, Krijnen P, Pieterman H et al. The effect of balloon angioplasty on hypertension in atherosclerotic renal-artery stenosis. Dutch Renal Artery Stenosis Intervention Cooperative Study Group. *N Engl J Med* 2000; **342**:1007–14.

59. Nordmann AJ, Woo K, Parkes R, Logan AG. Balloon angioplasty or medical therapy for hypertensive patients with atherosclerotic renal artery stenosis? A meta-analysis of randomized controlled trials. *Am J Med* 2003; **114**:44–50.

60. Creager MA, Jones DW, Easton JD et al. Atherosclerotic Vascular Disease Conference: Writing Group V: medical decision making and therapy. *Circulation* 2004; **109**:2634–42.

61. Watson PS, Hadjipetrou P, Cox SV, Piemonte TC, Eisenhauer AC. Effect of renal artery stenting on renal function and size in patients with atherosclerotic renovascular disease. *Circulation* 2000; **102**:1671–7.

62. Zeller T, Frank U, Muller C et al. Stent-supported angioplasty of severe atherosclerotic renal artery stenosis preserves renal function and improves blood pressure control: long-term results from a prospective registry of 456 lesions. *J Endovasc Ther* 2004; **11**:95–106.

63. Pickering TG, Herman L, Devereux RB et al. Recurrent pulmonary oedema in hypertension due to bilateral renal artery stenosis: treatment by angioplasty or surgical revascularisation. *Lancet* 1988; **2**:551–2.

64. Gray BH, Olin JW, Childs MB, Sullivan TM, Bacharach JM. Clinical benefit of renal artery angioplasty with stenting for the control of recurrent and refractory congestive heart failure. *Vasc Med* 2002; **7**:275–9.

65. Messina LM, Zelenock GB, Yao KA, Stanley JC. Renal revascularization for recurrent pulmonary edema in patients with poorly controlled hypertension and renal insufficiency: a distinct subgroup of patients with arteriosclerotic renal artery occlusive disease. *J Vasc Surg* 1992; **15**:73–80; discussion 80–2.

66. Pun E, Dowling RJ, Mitchell PJ. Acute presentations of renal artery stenosis in three patients with a solitary functioning kidney. *Australas Radiol* 2004; **48**:523–7.

67. Bax L, Mali WP, Buskens E et al. The benefit of STent placement and blood pressure and lipid-lowering for the prevention of progression of renal dysfunction caused by Atherosclerotic ostial stenosis of the Renal artery. The STAR-study: rationale and study design. *J Nephrol* 2003; **16**:807–12.

68. http://www.astral.bham.ac.uk.

69. http://www.clinicaltrials.gov.

70. Rocha-Singh K. Aortorenal artery translesion pressure gradients in renovascular hypertension: in search of clinical significance. *Catheter Cardiovasc Interven* 2003; **59**:378–9.

71. Rocha-Singh KJ, Mishkel GJ, Katholi RE et al. Clinical predictors of improved long-term blood pressure control after successful stenting of hypertensive patients with obstructive renal artery atherosclerosis. *Catheter Cardiovasc Interven* 1999; **47**:167–72.

72. Binkert CA, Hoffman U, Leung DA et al. Characterization of renal artery stenoses based on magnetic resonance renal flow and volume measurements. *Kidney Int* 1999; **56**:1846–54.

73. Tuttle KR. Renal parenchymal injury as a determinant of clinical consequences in atherosclerotic renal artery stenosis. *Am J Kidney Dis* 2002; **39**:1321–2.

74. Romero JC, Lerman LO. Novel noninvasive techniques for studying renal function in man. *Semin Nephrol* 2000; **20**:456–62.

75. Gerber BL, Ordoubadi FF, Wijns W et al. Positron emission tomography using (18)F-fluoro-deoxyglucose and euglycaemic hyperinsulinaemic glucose clamp: optimal criteria for the prediction of recovery of post-ischaemic left ventricular dysfunction. Results from the European Community Concerted Action Multicenter study on use of (18)F-fluoro-deoxyglucose Positron Emission Tomography for the Detection of Myocardial Viability. *Eur Heart J* 2001; **22**:1691–701.

76. Silva JA, Chan AW, White CJ et al. Elevated brain natriuretic peptide predicts blood pressure response after stent revascularization in patients with renal artery stenosis. *Circulation* 2005; **111**:328–33.

SECTION II

7. PREVENTION OF CONTRAST-INDUCED NEPHROPATHY WITH HYDRATION

Christian Müeller

Hydration remains the cornerstone for the prevention of contrast-induced nephropathy (CIN). It is safe, effective, and inexpensive.[1-7] Unfortunately, various important hydration details have not been well examined, including the timing and rate of the infusion and the respective values of intravenous and oral hydration. This chapter will try to address the following points:

- Effectiveness of hydration for CIN prevention;
- Route of administration;
- Type of saline solution;
- Hydration period, infusion rate and total hydration volume;
- Hydration in critical patients.

Pathogenesis of CIN

Both the pathogenesis of CIN in humans as well as the mechanisms of the preventive effect of hydration are incompletely understood. The pathogenesis of CIN seems to include renal vasoconstriction, medullary hypoxia, increased red cell aggregation, and direct toxic effects on renal epithelial cells.[3,8,9] Hydration results in plasma volume expansion with concomitant suppression of the renin–angiotensin–aldosterone system, downregulation of the tubuloglomerular feedback, dilution of the contrast media and thus prevention of renal cortical vasoconstriction, and avoidance of tubular obstruction.[3]

Since there seems to be no satisfactory animal model for CIN, it is likely that we will have to depend on more clinical intervention studies to further elucidate its pathophysiology.

Is hydration effective in the prevention of CIN?

For decades, the most honest answer to this pivotal questions was 'yes, probably'. Approximately 30 years ago, it was documented that dehydration accentuates the risk of CIN.[3,10] The incidence was higher in summer at a time when no special hydration was performed and patients were not allowed to drink before excretory urograms in order to maximize the concentration of contrast media in the urinary tract. Observations comparing hydrated patients with historic controls provided the first evidence that a fluid load might prevent CIN.[11-13] In 1994, these data were supported by a controlled study, primarily initiated to investigate the value of mannitol and furosemide administration.[1] In a randomized controlled trial including 78 patients with mild-to-moderate renal insufficiency, saline administration alone (0.45% saline over 24 hours starting 12 hours before administration of contrast media) was more effective than the combinations of hydration with mannitol (25 g given 1 hour before contrast media) or furosemide (80 mg iv).[1]

Recently, two randomized studies specifically examined the effectiveness of hydration. Trivedi and colleagues[5] randomized 53 patients on the day prior to scheduled elective cardiac catheterization to one of two groups: group 1 ($n = 27$) received normal saline for 24 hours (at a rate of 1 ml/kg per hour) beginning 12 hours prior to scheduled catheterization, and group 2 ($n = 26$) was allowed unrestricted oral fluids. Serum creatinine was measured 24 and 48 hours postcardiac catheterization and was compared to the prerandomization baseline value. The mean baseline calculated creatinine clearance was 80 μml/min and the mean baseline creatinine was 106 μmol/l. An increase in serum creatinine by at least 44.2 μmol/l (0.5 mg/dl), within 48 hours of contrast exposure, was considered to represent clinically significant acute renal failure. The incidence of acute renal failure was significantly lower in group 1 (1 out of 27) as compared to group 2 (9 out of 26; $P = 0.005$ for comparison between groups; relative risk 0.11, 95% confidence interval 0.02–0.79) (Figure 7.1). Bader and colleagues[6] randomized 39 patients with normal renal function receiving at least 80 ml of low-osmolarity contrast media during an angiographic procedure to one of the following hydration regimens: group 1 underwent volume expansion with 300 ml saline during contrast media administration ($n = 20$); group 2 received intravenous administration of at least 2000 ml saline within 12 hours before and after contrast media exposure ($n = 19$). Glomerular filtration rate (GFR) was measured by contrast media clearance (Renalyzer) at

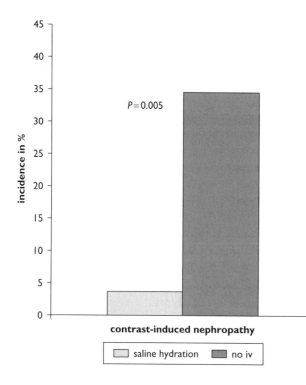

Figure 7.1 Saline hydration significantly reduces the risk of contrast-induced nephropathy.[5]

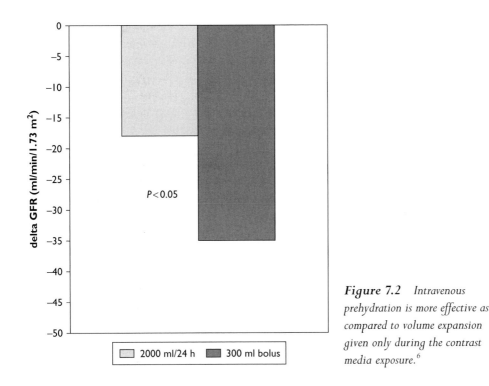

Figure 7.2 Intravenous prehydration is more effective as compared to volume expansion given only during the contrast media exposure.[6]

baseline and 48 hours after contrast media administration. The primary endpoint was the mean change in GFR after 48 hours. Patients in group 1 showed a significantly higher decline in GFR (Δ GFR 35 ml/min per 1.73 m^2) compared to patients receiving the intravenous prehydration regimen (Δ GFR 18 ml/min per 1.73 m^2; $P<0.05$) (Figure 7.2).

Therefore, the effectiveness of saline hydration is now well documented by observational as well as randomized studies. Since saline is cheap and safe, these data suggest that saline hydration should be considered in all patients undergoing investigations involving the use of intravenous or intra-arterial contrast media. This is especially true for patients with pre-existing risk factors for the development of contrast nephropathy.

Intravenous versus oral hydration

Until very recently, patients undergoing cardiac catheterization were kept nil by mouth to avoid vomiting and nausea, which was common with high-osmolality contrast agents, and to allow for tracheal intubation in case of failed percutaneous coronary intervention requiring emergency coronary artery bypass grafting. Although the strategy to keep the patient in a fasting state was well founded, many patients and physicians erroneously considered a restriction in fluids in parallel to the restriction in food. This misconception considerably impeded the widespread use of oral hydration prior to the contrast procedure.

Given the advances in both contrast agents and percutaneous interventional techniques, most institutions currently allow a light meal several hours ahead of cardiac catheterization. This change in management should encourage the use of oral fluids prior to cardiac catheterization and most of the other diagnostic procedures requiring intravenous contrast administration. Obviously, oral hydration is not an attractive option for patients undergoing abdominal CT-scanning who are receiving a high-volume oral fluid load to clean the bowel. Given their risk of dehydration from iatrogenic diarrhea, the intravenous infusion rate needs to be adapted.

Although 24-hour intravenous hydration with saline is highly effective in the prevention of contrast nephropathy, this regimen effectively precludes outpatient or 'same-day' contrast procedures. Despite this, economic pressures have increased the number of cardiac catheterizations in particular, and of contrast procedures in general, that are performed on the day of hospital admission. Therefore, an outpatient oral precatheterization hydration strategy has enormous appeal. Clinical data supporting this approach are scarce, but promising.

Taylor and colleagues[2] randomized 36 patients with mild-to-moderate renal dysfunction undergoing elective cardiac catheterization to receive either overnight in-hospital intravenous hydration (half-normal saline at 75 ml/hour for 12 hours before and 12 hours after catheterization; $n = 18$) or an outpatient hydration protocol including precatheterization oral hydration with 1000 ml water over 10 hours followed by 6 hours of intravenous hydration (half-normal saline at 300 ml/ hour) beginning 'on call' to the catheterization laboratory (30 to 60 minutes before exposure to contrast media). By protocol design, the outpatient group received a greater volume of hydration, although the net volume changes were comparable. The predefined primary endpoint, the maximal change in serum creatinine up to 48 hours after contrast exposure, was similar in both groups. Therefore, in conjunction with a 6-hour period of high-flow intravenous hydration started 30 to 60 minutes before the procedure, oral hydration seems to be a valuable option.

Moreover, a very low incidence of contrast nephropathy has been observed with the combination of intravenous hydration started with an infusion rate of 1 ml/kg of body weight per hour at 8 am on the day of percutaneous coronary intervention and strongly encouraged oral hydration (tea, mineral water).[4,14] Tea was provided to all patients in their room (500 ml) and in the post-PCI unit (at least 1000 ml) to encourage fluid intake.

What intravenous solution should be used for hydration?

Two intravenous solutions have been used predominantly in clinical practice and previous studies: normal isotonic (0.9%) saline and half-isotonic (0.45%) saline. Both solutions have been compared in a large trial. We have studied 1383 patients scheduled for elective or emergency coronary angioplasty.[4] Patients were randomly assigned to receive isotonic (0.9% saline) or half-isotonic (0.45% saline plus 5% glucose) hydration started in the morning of the procedure for elective interventions and immediately before for emergency interventions. Contrast nephropathy, defined as an increase in serum creatinine of at least 0.5 mg/dl (44 μmol/l) within 48 hours, was significantly reduced with isotonic (0.7% [95% CI, 0.1–1.4%]) versus half-isotonic hydration (2.0% [CI, 1.0–3.1%], $P = 0.04$) (Figure 7.3). Three predefined subgroups did benefit in particular from

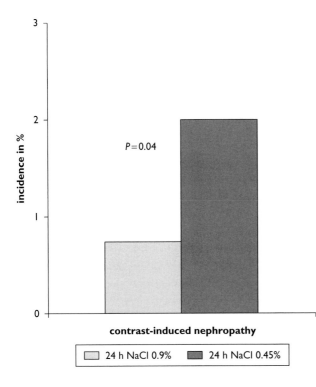

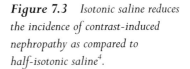

Figure 7.3 *Isotonic saline reduces the incidence of contrast-induced nephropathy as compared to half-isotonic saline[4].*

isotonic hydration: women, diabetics, and patients receiving more than 250 ml of contrast. Intravascular volume expansion at the critical time of contrast exposure seems to be the important element and is better accomplished by isotonic saline, which has a greater volume of distribution in the intravascular space compared to half-normal saline and unrestricted oral fluids, the latter being likely to be less than isotonic.

Based on the hypothesis that alkalizing renal tubular fluid with bicarbonate may reduce free radical formation and thus reduce injury, Merten and colleagues evaluated an alternative hydration protocol with sodium bicarbonate.[15] A total of 119 patients with pre-existing renal insufficiency who were scheduled mainly for cardiac catheterization were randomized to receive either 154 mEq/l sodium bicarbonate or equiosmolar sodium chloride (saline), both given as an intravenous bolus (3 ml/kg per hour for 1 hour) immediately before administration of iopamidol, followed by an infusion at a rate of 1 ml/kg per hour for 6 hours after the procedure. The incidence of CIN (defined as an increase of $\geq 25\%$ of baseline serum creatinine within 2 days) was lower in the bicarbonate group (1.7% vs 13.6%; $P = 0.02$) (Figure 7.4). These interesting results are hampered by the fact that a 7-hour instead of a 24-hour hydration period was used, which does not allow direct comparison with previous studies. Therefore, further studies are required to elucidate the role of sodium bicarbonate in the prevention of CIN. Currently, both normal saline and bicarbonate can be justified as the primary hydration solution.

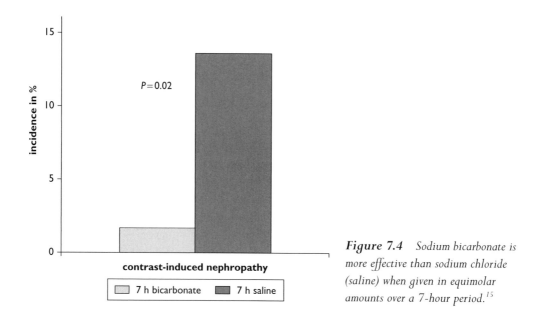

Figure 7.4 *Sodium bicarbonate is more effective than sodium chloride (saline) when given in equimolar amounts over a 7-hour period.[15]*

Hydration period, infusion rate, and total hydration volume

Unfortunately, we lack data from controlled clinical trials that define the most effective hydration period, infusion rate, or hydration volume. Rather than effectiveness, feasibility and safety have had a major impact on the regimens that are used in clinical practice.

Feasibility

Intravenous hydration requires placement of a venous catheter and starting an infusion several hours ahead of the contrast procedure. This at times causes logistic problems, even in elective in-hospital patients, and significantly limits the use of hydration for emergency procedures or outpatients.

Safety

High infusion rate or high total hydration volume may result in volume overload and trigger pulmonary edema in patients with predisposing cardiac conditions. Given the considerable overlap between patients at high risk for CIN and patients with cardiac disease and risk for pulmonary edema, this concern is very real. As a result, a rather low infusion rate of 1 ml/kg per hour has in general been recommended and used in clinical practice. We have learned from controlled trials that a saline bolus of 300 ml given during the procedure is significantly inferior to 2000 ml given over a 24-hour hydration period.[6] On the other hand, if accompanied with oral prehydration, a very high infusion rate of 300 ml per hour begun 'on call' to the catheterization laboratory (30 to 60 minutes before exposure to contrast media) and continued for a total of 6 hours was equally effective as a standard 24-hour protocol with an infusion rate of 75 ml per hour.

In summary, whenever logistics permit, a 24-hour protocol with 1 ml/kg per hour begun 12 hours before the procedure (or at least in the morning of the procedure[4]) should be implemented. Using a high infusion rate of 300 ml per hour–at least for the first hour[15]–seems to be an effective alternative, if the infusion can be started 1 hour prior to contrast exposure.

Hydration for the prevention of CIN in patients in the intensive care unit

CIN has been defined as an acute decline in renal function following the administration of intravenous (or intra-arterial) contrast media in the absence of other causes. As critically ill patients in general nearly always do have other potential causes for an acute decline in renal function, a strict separation of this clinical entity is difficult in the setting of intensive care. Arterial hypovolemia and impaired renal perfusion are very common in critically ill patients and represent detrimental comorbidities with respect to CIN.[16] Therefore, adequate hydration is of paramount importance and a *sine qua non* in critically ill patients scheduled for contrast procedures. It is important to note that, in general, both the infusion rate and total infusion volume necessary to adequately hydrate a critically ill patient by far exceed those used in elective patients. Obviously, patients in pulmonary edema or cardiogenic shock are an important exception to this rule.

Conclusions

Hydration remains the cornerstone for the prevention of CIN. Current evidence suggests that the combination of intravenous and oral hydration effectively prevents CIN in low- and moderate-risk patients. Normal isotonic (0.9%) saline should be started 12 hours before (or at least in the morning of) the contrast procedure with an infusion rate of 1 ml/kg of body weight per hour and should be continued for 24 hours. In addition, patients should be encouraged to drink plenty of fluids (tea, mineral water). The use of bicarbonate infusion may allow shorter hydration periods. Combined intravenous and oral hydration protocols limiting the intravenous infusion to the contrast procedure period have been designed for outpatients and are under investigation. In summary, in view of the evident effectiveness of hydration as a CIN preventive strategy, additional research should continue to define further details regarding its optimal use in patients receiving contrast media.

Acknowledgment

Dr Mueller was supported by research grants from the Swiss National Science Foundation, the Swiss Heart Foundation, the Novartis Foundation, the University of Basel, Abbott, Biosite, Bracco, Roche, and Schering.

References

1. Solomon R, Werner C, Mann D, D'Elia J, Silva P. Effects of saline, mannitol, and furosemide on acute decrease in renal function induced by radiocontrast agents. *N Engl J Med* 1994; **331**:1416–20.

2. Taylor AJ, Hotchkiss D, Morse RW, McCabe J. PREPARED: Preparation for angiography in renal dysfunction. A randomized trial of inpatient versus outpatient hydration protocols for cardiac catheterization in mild to moderate renal dysfunction. *Chest* 1998; **114**:1570–4.

3. Erley CM. Does hydration prevent radiocontrast-induced acute renal failure? *Nephrol Dial Transplant* 1999; **14**:1064–6.

4. Mueller C, Buerkle G, Buettner HJ et al. Prevention of contrast media-associated nephropathy: randomized comparison of two hydration regimens in 1620 patients undergoing coronary angioplasty. *Arch Intern Med* 2002; **162**:329–36.

5. Trivedi HS, Moore H, Nasr S et al. A randomized prospective trial to assess the role of saline hydration on the development of contrast nephropathy. *Nephron Clin Pract* 2003; **93**:c29–c34.

6. Bader BD, Berger ED, Heede MB et al. What is the best hydration regimen to prevent contrast media-induced nephrotoxicity? *Clin Nephrol* 2004; **62**:1–7.

7. Holt S. Radiocontrast media-induced renal injury – saline is effective in prevention. *Nephron Clin Pract* 2003; **93**:c5–c6.

8. Heyman SN, Rosen S, Brezis M. Radiocontrast nephropathy: a paradigm for the synergism between toxic and hypoxic insults in the kidney. *Exp Nephrol* 1994; **2**:153–7.

9. Maeder M, Klein M, Fehr T, Rickli H. Contrast nephropathy: review focusing on prevention. *J Am Coll Cardiol* 2004; **44**:1763–71.

10. Byrd L, Sherman RL. Radiocontrast-induced acute renal failure: a clinical and pathological review. *Medicine* 1979; **58**:270–9.

11. Anto HR, Chou SY, Porush JG et al. Infusion intravenous pyelography and renal function. Effect of hypertonic mannitol in patients with chronic renal insufficiency. *Arch Intern Med* 1981; **141**:1652–6.

12. Eisenberg RL, Blank WO, Hedgock MW. Renal failure after major angiography can be avoided with hydration. *Am J Radiol* 1981; **136**:859–61.

13. Kerstein MD, Puyau FA. Value of preangiography hydration. *Surgery* 1984; **96**:919–22.

14. Mueller C, Buerkle G, Perruchoud AP, Buettner HJ. Female sex and the risk of contrast nephropathy after percutaneous coronary intervention. *Can J Cardiol* 2004; **20**:505–10.

15. Merten GJ, Burgess WP, Gray LV et al. Prevention of contrast-induced nephropathy with sodium bicarbonate. A randomized controlled trial. *JAMA* 2004; **291**:2328–34.

16. Ronco C, Bellomo R. Prevention of acute renal failure in the critically ill. *Nephron Clin Pract* 2003; **93**:c13–c20.

8. CONTRAST MEDIA: PHYSICOCHEMIC PROPERTIES, PHYSIOLOGIC EFFECTS, AND SELECTION

Roxana Mehran, Robert Siegel, and Eugenia Nikolsky

Introduction

Routine medical practice includes frequent use of radiocontrast agents for both diagnostic and therapeutic purposes. Despite efforts to improve the safety of existing contrast agents, all can cause adverse reactions that range from mild to severe and even life-threatening.

This chapter discusses the currently available contrast agents, their physical, chemical and physiologic properties, as well as adverse effects associated with their use. The chapter concludes with a review of major clinical trials that have assessed different contrast agents, along with recommendations for cost-effective strategies to select the optimal agent for individual patients. The following discussion applies only to water-soluble, intravenous, iodinated agents used with X-rays. Water-insoluble (barium) and 'oily' contrast agents, as well as contrast agents used in magnetic resonance imaging and ultrasound, are beyond the scope of this discussion.

Physicochemical properties

The iodine atom has an atomic weight of 120.90;[1] its large nucleus attenuates X-ray beams much more effectively than the nuclei of the carbon, hydrogen, nitrogen, and oxygen atoms that mainly comprise most non-bony human tissue. Administration of iodine-rich compounds into an anatomic space therefore makes that space appear brighter than most surrounding tissues on X-ray imaging. This effect persists until the iodine-containing molecules have mostly diffused away from the anatomic space.

The iodine-containing agents employed to create transient high-contrast images have varying physicochemical properties, and can be classified by the iodine content (quantity of iodine per ml of solution), osmolarity (hyperosmolar vs low-osmolar vs iso-osmolar), level of ionization (ionic vs non-ionic), and degree of polymerization (monomeric vs dimeric) (Table 8.1). The structure of currently used agents is based on the fully substituted benzoic acid with three iodine atoms at positions 2, 4, and 6 on the benzene ring. In its simplest form, tri-iodinated benzoic acid, the benzene ring is anionic and hyperosmolar (Figure 8.1(a)). Adding hydroxyl groups or other hydrophilic conjugates to the molecule allows the creation of non-ionic agents and can reduce the agent's osmolarity. The following categories of water-soluble intravascular iodinated agents are commonly used:

Table 8.1   Physicochemic properties of commonly used water-soluble intravascular iodinated radiocontrast agents

Compound	Trade name	Polymerization	Ionization	Osmolality mOsm/ kg H₂O	Viscosity cP @20°C	cP @37°C	Iodine mg/ml
Diatrizoate	Reno-Cal-76®	Monomeric	Ionic	1870	15*	9.1	370
Iohexol	Omnipaque® 350	Monomeric	Non-ionic	844	20.4	10.4	350
Iopamidol	Isovue® 370	Monomeric	Non-ionic	796	20.9	9.4	370
Ioversol	Opitray® 350	Monomeric	Non-ionic	792	18	9.0	350
Ioxaglate	Hexabrix® 320	Dimeric	Ionic	600	15.7	7.5	320
Iodixanol	Visipaque® 320	Dimeric	Non-ionic	290	26.6	11.8	320

*@25°C

Reno-Cal-76® and Isovue®: Bracco Diagnostics Inc. Princeton, NJ, USA;
Omnipaque® 350 and Visipaque® 320: Amersham Health Princeton, NJ, USA;
Optiray® 350: Mallinckrodt Inc. St. Louis, MO, USA;
Hexabrix® 320: Mallinckrodt Inc. St. Louis, MO, USA (under licence from Guerbet Roissy, France).

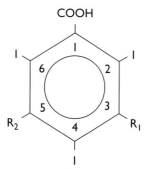

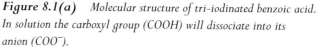

Figure 8.1(a)   *Molecular structure of tri-iodinated benzoic acid. In solution the carboxyl group (COOH) will dissociate into its anion (COO⁻).*

Ionic monomers.   Often called 'conventional' agents, these compounds have high osmolarity – up to seven times higher than plasma osmolarity. They contain three iodine atoms for every two molecules produced in solution. Ionic monomers have high concentrations of cations – mostly sodium – along with the iodine-containing anions. These are among the oldest and generally least expensive of the water-soluble iodinated contrast agents used extensively in clinical practice. Examples include iothalamate and diatrizoate (Figure 8.1(b)).

Non-ionic monomers.   These substances do not ionize into an anion and a cation, effectively cutting the particle number in half for any iodine concentration compared to the ionic monomers. Osmolarity depends on the number of molecules per unit volume of solution; the lower number of particles makes these agents 'low-osmolarity' compared to 'conventional' contrast. These formulations, often called 'non-ionic' and 'low-osmolar' agents, each contain three iodine atoms per

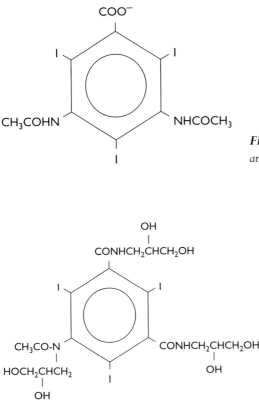

Figure 8.1(b) Molecular structure of diatrizoate, an ionic monomer.

Figure 8.1(c) Molecular structure of iohexol, a non-ionic monomer.

molecule. Iohexol (Figure 8.1(c)), iopamidol, iopromide, ioversol, and ioxilan are members of this category.

Ionic dimers. Like the ionic monomers, these agents consist of a cation (predominantly sodium) and an iodine-containing anion. The anion is a dimer that contains six iodine atoms. When the ionic complex dissociates, it creates two particles: a cation with no iodine, and an anion with six iodine atoms. The net effect is a compound with a ratio of three iodine atoms for every molecule in solution, yielding a similar osmolarity to the non-ionic monomers. Ioxaglate (Figure 8.1(d)) is the only commercially available contrast agent in this category.

Non-ionic dimers. Combining the non-dissociating properties of the non-ionic monomers with the dimeric properties of the ionic dimers allows these substances to achieve even lower osmolarity. Each molecule in this family has six iodine atoms. The molecule does not dissociate in solution. Iodixanol (Figure 8.1(e)) and iotrilan are members of this family, frequently referred to as 'iso-osmolar' agents. Iotrilan is nearly iso-osmolar to plasma (0.32 osm/kg H_2O), while iodixanol is hypo-osmolar (0.29 osm/kg H_2O); some commercially available forms of these agents include sodium and calcium salts added to increase the liquid's osmolarity.

   These newer agents have larger molecules than older agents; as the molecules increase in size, the contrast medium becomes more viscous.

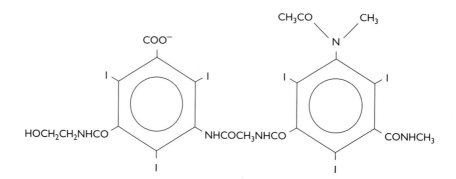

Figure 8.1(d) *Molecular structure of ioxaglate, an ionic dimer.*

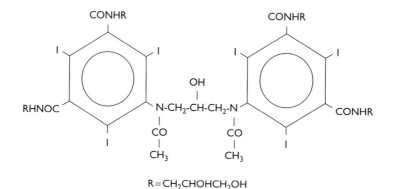

Figure 8.1(e) *Molecular structure of iodixanol, a non-ionic dimer.*

Physiologic effects

Pharmacokinetics

Different contrast media share similar pharmacokinetics.[2-5] Following intravascular infusion, the agents mix into the circulating plasma volume while simultaneously passing freely across normal blood vessel walls into the extravascular extracellular space. These compounds remain almost entirely unbound to proteins. They do not enter cells to any significant degree and do not cross a normal, intact blood–brain barrier. The volume of distribution is approximately 165 ml/kg, and elimination proceeds by first-order pharmacokinetics with a half-life of approximately 2 hours.

Renal excretion. In patients with preserved renal function, the discussed contrast agents are primarily excreted by passive glomerular filtration, with no significant tubular excretion or reabsorption. During excretion the distal and collecting tubules resorb water from the tubular space, concentrating the contrast in the tubular filtrate. This water resorption during excretion depends

108

on vasopressin levels (antidiuretic hormone [ADH]) in the distal and collecting tubules.[6,7] The presence of contrast agents in the tubular filtrate antagonizes these renal concentrating mechanisms; this effect occurs more with higher osmolarity agents.

Kidneys with normal function can generate high urine concentrations of the contrast agents. Because of their predominantly renal excretion, contrast agents have been successfully used to measure the glomerular filtration rate (GFR) by infusing intravenous contrast, then taking serial measurements of contrast agent plasma concentration.[8]

Other physiologic excretion.   Liver uptake of ionic monomers may reach up to 5% of an administered dose, but hepatic uptake of the other agents is trivial in the presence of normal renal function.[9] In patients with endstage renal disease (ESRD), the liver becomes the most important, albeit slow, physiologic route of excretion for all the agents. Trace amounts (less than 2%) of all agents are routinely excreted in sweat, tears, and saliva.[9]

Hemodialysis.   The molecular weight of different iodinated contrast agents ranges between 800 and 1200 Da, making contrast media readily dialyzable. The plasma clearance of most modern contrast media is 50 to 70 ml/min, with more than 80% of the agent removed from the plasma pool in 4–5 hours of hemodialysis.[10] (These data are based on a hemodialysis blood flow of 200 ml/min and a dialysate of 500 ml/min.) Non-ionic monomers are cleared more rapidly than the dimers, presumably because of their smaller molecular size.[11] Hemodialysis does not protect poorly functioning kidneys against contrast-induced nephropathy.[12,13]

Pregnancy and lactation

During human pregnancy, the safety of administering iodinated contrast media remains unclear. Animal studies have failed to demonstrate harmful effects of contrast media with respect to the reproduction, development of the embryo or fetus, course of gestation, or peri- and postnatal development with doses of contrast agents greater than 100 times the human dose.[14,15] However, other iodine-containing organic preparations administered near term have caused hypothyroidism in some human neonates.[16] Because radiation exposure should be avoided during pregnancy when possible, the benefits of a radiographic examination, with or without contrast, should be weighed against potential risks.

Contrast media are minimally excreted in human breast milk and are poorly absorbed by the intestine. Harm to the nursing infant is therefore unlikely, but safety has not been established in clinical trials. Current guidelines recommend abstaining from breast feeding for at least 24 hours after contrast administration.

Adverse effects

Water-soluble X-ray contrast agents have uncommonly low toxicity. However, they are used in extraordinarily high concentrations and total doses. During a computed tomography examination 30 g of iodine may be injected intravenously within 30 seconds. During some percutaneous interventional procedures clinicians commonly administer more than four times this total dose. In these doses, the hyperosmolarity of the solution causes non-specific hydrophobic interactions with structural and functional proteins, leading to unusual toxic effects. These osmotically induced

Table 8.2 Adverse effects of contrast agents in specific conditions

Predisposing condition	Adverse effect
Renal insufficiency, diabetes mellitus, hypovolemia, nephrotoxins, and advanced age	Contrast-induced nephropathy
End-stage renal disease (ESRD)	Neurotoxicity
Pulmonary hypertension or severe heart failure	Hypervolemia
Allergy or asthma	Allergic reaction/anaphylaxis
Sickle cell disease	Hemolysis/sickle crisis
Pheochromocytoma	Hypertensive crisis
Hyperthyroidism	Thyrotoxicosis
Radioiodine thyroid ablation	Ablation failure

side-effects occur in addition to the standard chemotoxic effects seen with any drug. A number of specific conditions are associated with a predisposition to toxic reactions to contrast agents (Table 8.2);

- Renal insufficiency
- Diabetes mellitus
- Hypovolemia
- Concurrent administration of nephrotoxic drugs and
- Advanced age

all predispose toward contrast-induced nephropathy. (Please refer to other chapters in this book for further information.)

Endstage renal disease (ESRD): neurotoxicity.   In patients with ESRD and anuria, renal toxicity *per se* is not an issue given the pre-exposure irreversible damage of renal function. The issue then becomes whether the retained contrast may exert toxic effects on other organ systems. Contrast agents may potentially damage the blood–brain barrier and exert neurotoxic effects. Several case reports demonstrated acute reversible neurologic changes associated with administration.[17–20] Other adverse reactions reported in patients with ESRD include skin disorders, vasculitis, and salivary gland swelling.[11]

   Although local clinical practice in many institutions involves performing hemodialysis promptly after contrast administration to reduce the risk of toxic effect, scientific investigations have not provided evidence to support this approach. Additionally, toxic events occur predominantly within minutes of contrast administration,[10,21] i.e. before hemodialysis could remove a significant amount

Table 8.3   Symptoms of hypersensitivity reactions to contrast agents

Category	Symptoms
Common allergic	Angioedema, chill, choking, conjunctivitis, coughing, diaphoresis, edema, fever, headache, hoarseness, nausea, rhinitis, sneezing, wheezing
Cutaneous	Erythema multiforme minor, urticaria, flushing, rash, dermatitis, skin eruptions, pruritus, toxic epidermal necrolysis
Gastrointestinal	Emesis
Cardiovascular and hemodynamic	Hypertension, hypotension, cardiac arrhythmias, cardiac arrest
Respiratory	Tachypnea, dyspnea, bronchospasm, asthma attack, cyanosis, pulmonary infiltration, respiratory arrest
Vegetative/neural	Chest, low back and lumbar pain, confusion, sensation of warmth, tingling, panic of imminent death
Delayed (days)	Generalized maculopapular exanthema

Adapted from Szebeni J[23].

of contrast. Based on these data, published clinical guidelines have stated that correlation of timing of contrast agent injection with hemodialysis is not beneficial, and that extra hemodialysis sessions for removal of the contrast are not necessary.[22]

Pulmonary hypertension or heart failure (severe): hypervolemia.   The volume-expanding effect of contrast agents increases preload, which may further increase pulmonary artery and venous pressures. We recommend minimizing the volume of contrast agent in these patients, performing periprocedure hemodynamic monitoring using a Swan–Ganz catheter, and considering prompt hemodialysis after contrast administration.

Allergy or asthma: allergic reaction/anaphylaxis.   Contrast media are well known to cause hypersensitivity reactions, ranging from mild symptoms to severe anaphylactoid reactions (Table 8.3).[23] The pathophysiology involves multiple mechanisms, including complement-mediated pathways, IgE-mediated degranulation of mast cells and basophils, direct secretory effects on mast cells and basophils due to local changes in osmolarity and ion concentrations, and activation of plasma proteolytic systems. Non-acute delayed-type hypersensitivity reactions have also been reported.[24]

Three large observational studies indicated that immediate, mild adverse reactions occur in 3.8 to 12.7% of patients receiving intravenous injections of high-osmolar, ionic agents and in

0.7–3.1% of patients receiving low-osmolar non-ionic agents.[25–27] Severe immediate reactions have been reported to occur with a frequency of 0.1 to 0.4% for ionic agents and with a frequency of 0.02 to 0.04% for non-ionic agents.[25–28] Although the adverse reactions observed with the non-ionic agents are usually less severe than the reactions induced by the ionic agents, the death rates for the two types of products are not significantly different, with a mortality rate estimated to occur in 1 of 100 000 examinations.[28]

Although hypersensitivity reactions can occur in patients without a history of atopy, prior symptoms of allergy or asthma are associated with an elevated risk of hypersensitivity reaction to contrast media. Skin testing is not a reliable predictor of hypersensitivity reactions to contrast agents.[24] Main factors influencing the severity of contrast media reactions include rate of administration, amount of contrast infused, and type of contrast agent used. When patients with a previous reaction to an ionic contrast medium are subsequently given a non-ionic contrast agent, an up to 10-fold reduction in the incidence of severe repeat reactions has been reported.[29] Prophylactic administration of corticosteroids and antihistamines may reduce the incidence and severity of allergic reactions, however this practice does not totally eliminate the risk of contrast-induced anaphylactic reactions.[24]

Sickle cell disease: hemolysis/sickle crisis Iodinated radiographic contrast media have traditionally been relatively contraindicated in patients with sickle cell disease because their high osmolality may induce osmotic shrinkage of red blood cells, impair blood flow through the microcirculation, and precipitate or exacerbate a sickle cell crisis. Contrast agents may cause shrinkage of the red blood cells and produce 'dessicocytes', or change their shape, producing 'echinocytes' or 'stomatocytes'. Dessicocyte formation is proportional to the concentration and osmolality of the contrast agent, while echinocyte and stomatocyte formation is dependent on the chemotoxicity of the agent. While dessicocytes are seen more often with agents at higher osmolality, all contrast agents induce the same degree of echinocyte formation, and stomatocytes are seen more often with the iso-osmolal, non-ionic dimers[30–33]. The combined effect of changes in morphology is reduced plasticity of the red blood cells and decrease in blood flow through the capillaries. An *in vitro* study has evaluated the effect of various contrast agents on red cell morphology, hematology, and red cell flow resistance through a micropore filter. Blood was tested from 10 normal and 10 sickle cell donors at contrast agent concentrations of 0, 1, 10, and 30% weight/volume in an attempt to approximate the relative concentrations of contrast medium to blood that might occur during the bolus-injection and circulation-diluted phases of contrast agent administration. Contrast agents tested were a high-osmolar ionic agent, two low-osmolar agents, and the iso-osmolar iodixanol. All contrast media had minor effects on red blood cell morphology. Cases of blindness[35] and stroke[36] have been reported in patients with hemoglobin sickle cell (SS) disease after contrast administration. There are also case reports of hemolysis following contrast administration in patients with SS disease.[37,38]

Pheochromocytoma: hypertensive crisis. Contrast media administration is known to cause severe hypertension in patients with pheochromocytoma.[39] Blood pressure should be monitored during contrast administration. Most authors recommend minimization of the amount of contrast used; the value of pretreatment with alpha-blocking agents is controversial.[39,40]

Hyperthyroidism: thyrotoxicosis. Contrast agent administration has been shown to induce thyroid storm in hyperthyroid patients.[39] Iodine-induced thyrotoxicosis may occur 4 to 12 weeks after

Table 8.4 Effects of contrast on laboratory testing

Diagnostic test	Contrast-induced abnormalities
Thyroid	
Serum thyroid function testing	Altered protein-bound iodine levels
Radioactive iodine scans	Altered thyroid uptake
Hematologic	
Blood cell counts	Transiently decreased
Prothrombin time	Transiently increased
Thromboplastin time	Transiently increased
Basic metabolic profile	
Sodium	Hyponatremia
Potassium	Hyperkalemia
Bicarbonate	Metabolic acidosis
Urine chemistries	
All quantitative urine chemistry analysis	Altered concentrations of urine chemicals

contrast injection, and elderly patients may be more sensitive to the effect of contrast media on thyroid function. Prophylactic administration of perchlorate, thiamazole, or both in high-risk patients with hyperthyroidism has been recommended.[41] In euthyroid patients, thyrotoxicosis after contrast administration is rare,[42] but may occur more commonly in elderly patients.[43] See also 'Effects on laboratory testing' below.

Radioiodine thyroid ablation: ablation failure.   Potentially, the iodine atoms in the contrast media may thwart an effort to perform radioiodine thyroid ablation. Current recommendations advise avoiding use of iodinated contrast for 2 months prior to ablative therapy.[41]

Homocystinuria: thrombosis and embolism.   Although many contrast manufacturers warn of possible thrombosis or embolism in patients with homocystinuria, no published case reports have confirmed the existence of this phenomenon.

Effects on laboratory testing

Known effects of contrast administration on laboratory tests are summarized in Table 8.4.

Thyroid function testing and thyroid imaging.   Intravascular administration of iodinated contrast may alter serum protein-bound iodine concentrations and radioactive iodine or pertechnetate ion uptake for up to 2 weeks. Other thyroid function tests not dependent on measurement of iodine, such as resin triiodothyronine (RTI) uptake, may not be affected.[41]

Urinalysis.   In the presence of normal renal function, very high urine concentrations of contrast may be achieved. The non-ionic dimers have even been found to achieve original bottle-strength concentration in the urine.[44] The presence of high concentrations of contrast in the urine in the 48 hours after contrast administration interferes with chemical testing of the urine.

Basic metabolic profile. Serum chemistry testing shortly after contrast administration may show a decrease in sodium and bicarbonate concentrations and an increase in potassium concentration;[45] the hyponatremia has been implicated in cases of neurologic damage.[46]

Hematologic testing. Leukocyte and erythrocyte counts may be transiently decreased. *In vitro* tests with animal blood have demonstrated slight inhibition of all stages of coagulation with contrast media; prothrombin time and thromboplastin time may increase after administration of contrast agents.[47]

Contrast agent selection

This section includes a review of data comparing the physiologic effects of different contrast agents, followed by summaries of the major studies that have compared the toxicities of different contrast agents.

Differences between contrast agents in experimental studies and animal models

In animal models, high-osmolar contrast agents have been shown to cause more prominent cytotoxic effects,[48,49] greater enzymuria,[50] and greater decreases in glomerular filtration rate[51] and creatinine clearance[52] compared to low-osmolar contrast media. However, histologic studies failed to detect significant differences in the degree of renal damage using contrast agents with different osmolarities.[53]

When the effect of contrast media on cortical, inner medullary, and outer medullary blood flow of the rat kidney was investigated by means of laser-Doppler flowmetry, the high-osmolar contrast agent diatrizoate and the low-osmolar contrast agents ioxaglate and iobitridol appeared to produce similar changes. Neither agent significantly modified medullary perfusion, but each of them decreased the cortical blood flow.[54] However, iodixanol induced a dose-dependent reduction of perfusion in all examined regions. Moreover, reducing viscosity by warming the contrast solution alleviated the reduction of inner medullary and cortical blood flow induced by iodixanol, a relatively high-viscosity contrast agent. This suggests that reduced viscosity may palliate the detrimental effects of iodixanol on the inner medulla and the cortex.[54]

Quantitative endothelial cell injury in a rat model, assessed by autoradiography, has been reported to be significantly less after exposure to non-ionic contrast agent (iomeprol) compared with ionic contrast material (ioxithalamate).[55] On the other hand, the ionic dimer ioxaglate, compared with the non-ionic dimer iodixanol, has been shown to cause less prominent hypoperfusion and hypoxia in the outer medullary region of the kidney in dogs.[56] Moreover, different effects of contrast agents on endothelial and smooth muscle cell growth have been demonstrated *in vitro*. A study in cultured bovine aortic endothelial and smooth muscle cells exposed to ionic (iothalamate) or non-ionic (ioversol or iopamidol) contrast agents showed an alteration in structure and a decrease in proliferation lasting for up to 7 days.[57] In this study the ionic contrast agent induced more severe changes in endothelial cells, while the non-ionic contrast agent had more pronounced effects on smooth muscle cells.

Scheller et al examined the influence of several types of contrast media on rheologic parameters of blood in humans. In this study, exposure to both ionic and non-ionic contrast media resulted in a similar decrease in plasma viscosity, erythrocyte aggregation, and platelet reactivity index, while the decrease in hematocrit was significantly greater following the use of an ionic agent.[58] In a double-blind clinical study by Tschakert et al in 50 patients with normal renal function, the degree of enzymuria was significantly less when ionic rather than non-ionic contrast was used.[59]

Early clinical data: the 1993 radiology meta-analysis[60]

Authors searched for randomized trials that compared low-osmolarity contrast media to higher-osmolarity media and that collected data on changes in glomerular filtration rate or serum creatinine levels. They performed a meta-analysis on the 24 trials in which they found adequate available data. They reported that a pooled odds risk of an increase in serum creatinine of more than 0.5 mg/dl with a low-osmolarity contrast was 0.61 (95% confidence interval [CI] 0.48–0.77) times the odds seen with high-osmolarity contrast. Within the subgroup of patients with existing renal insufficiency, this odds ratio was 0.5 (CI 0.36–0.68), while it was 0.75 (CI 0.52–1.1) in the subgroup with normal renal function. Greater increases in serum creatinine occurred only in patients with existing renal failure; these increases were observed less commonly with low-osmolarity contrast (odds ratio, 0.44; CI 0.26–0.73).

Ionic monomers, non-ionic monomers, and risk factors for contrast-induced nephropathy: the Iohexol Cooperative study

Investigators performed a randomized, double-blind, prospective, multicenter controlled trial to compare the toxicities of diatrizoate, an ionic monomer, to iohexol, a non-ionic monomer.[61] They stratified 1390 clinically stable patients undergoing cardiac angiography into groups according to the presence of diabetes mellitus and level of serum creatinine. They randomized subjects to receive either diatrizoate or iohexol, and tabulated all adverse events that occurred during and immediately after angiography. Significant differences were found in the number of patients with contrast-media-related adverse events (iohexol vs diatrizoate: 10.2 vs 31.6%; $P < 0.001$) and cardiac adverse events (7.2 vs 24.5%; $P < 0.001$). Severe reactions and the need for treatment were more frequent with diatrizoate than with iohexol, but there was no difference in the incidence of death. The presence of New York Heart Association classification 3 or 4 and serum creatinine greater than or equal to 1.5 mg/dl at baseline predicted a higher incidence of adverse events after angiography.

A subsequent analysis investigated risk of developing contrast-induced nephropathy.[62] Patients were stratified into four groups: renal insufficiency and diabetes mellitus both absent ($n = 364$); renal insufficiency absent, diabetes mellitus present ($n = 318$); renal insufficiency present, diabetes mellitus absent ($n = 298$); and renal insufficiency and diabetes mellitus both present ($n = 216$). Serum creatinine levels were measured before and after coronary angiography. Prophylactic hydration was administered before and after the procedure. Acute nephrotoxicity, which the authors defined as an increase in serum creatinine of greater than or equal to 1 mg/dl 48 to 72 hours post-contrast, was reported in 42 (7%) patients who received diatrizoate compared to 19 (3%) patients

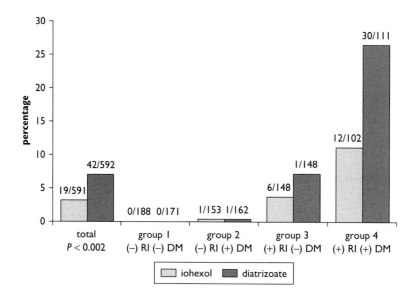

Figure 8.2 *Incidence of contrast-induced nephropathy, stratified by diabetes mellitus (DM) and chronic renal insufficiency (RI): data from the Iohexol Cooperative study. The bars show the percentage of patients with an increase in serum creatinine of greater than or equal to 1 mg/dl at 48 or 72 hours after contrast administration. (From Rudnik et al.[59]).*

who received iohexol, with a *P* value less than 0.002. Differences in nephrotoxicity between the two contrast groups were confined to patients with renal insufficiency alone or combined with diabetes mellitus. Patients with renal insufficiency receiving diatrizoate were 3.3 times more likely to develop acute nephrotoxicity compared to those receiving iohexol.

Virtually no patients with normal baseline renal function developed acute nephrotoxicity in this study, regardless of contrast agent used. Diabetes alone did not pose a significant predisposition to contrast-induced nephropathy, but renal failure with diabetes was associated with an increased risk of nephropathy compared to renal failure without diabetes (Figure 8.2).

These results were corroborated in a randomized study by Taliercio et al of 307 patients with baseline renal insufficiency (serum creatinine ≥ 1.5 mg/dl), in which the degree of renal function deterioration was less with the non-ionic agent iopamidol than with the ionic agent diatrizoate as measured by the mean of the maximal increase in serum creatinine (0.20 ± 0.44 vs 0.38 ± 0.73 mg/dl, $P < 0.0001$) and the incidence of contrast-induced nephropathy (defined as an increase in serum creatinine > 0.5 mg/dl) (8% versus 19%, $P < 0.01$).[63] On the other hand, a 443-patient randomized study by Schwab et al failed to show a significant difference in the rates of CIN in the group exposed to iopamidol versus diatrizoate, either in low- or high-risk patients.[64]

Non-ionic monomers vs non-ionic dimers in patients with renal insufficiency: the NEPHRIC study

Whether the iso-osmolar agent iodixanol is less nephrotoxic than other low-osmolar contrast media has been recently studied. Chalmers and Jackson could not find a significantly reduced incidence of

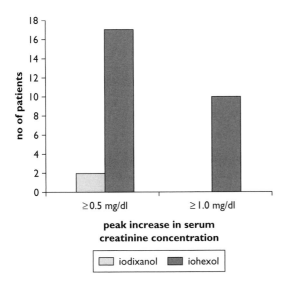

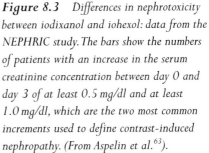

Figure 8.3 *Differences in nephrotoxicity between iodixanol and iohexol: data from the NEPHRIC study. The bars show the numbers of patients with an increase in the serum creatinine concentration between day 0 and day 3 of at least 0.5 mg/dl and at least 1.0 mg/dl, which are the two most common increments used to define contrast-induced nephropathy. (From Aspelin et al.[63]).*

CIN with iodixanol vs iohexol in an unblinded study of 104 patients with baseline renal insufficiency[65]. In this trial, the incidence of CIN was 3.7% with iodixanol (the iso-osmolar group) and 10.0% with iohexol (the low-osmolar group, p = n.s.). Two other small studies also found no difference in nephrotoxicity with iodixanol compared to low-osmolar agents in patients with chronic renal insufficiency[66,67] except for the high-osmolar agent, which caused marked echinocytosis and reduced filterability. Filterability effects were greater for sickle cells than for normal red cells. Another *in vitro* study found that non-ionic contrast induced less sickling than ionic contrast[34]. These results suggest that the use of non-ionic contrast agents may reduce the risk of contrast-induced sickle crisis.

To further compare iodixanol and iohexol, the Nephrotoxicity in High-Risk Patients Study of Iso-Osmolar and Low-Osmolar Non-Ionic Contrast Media (NEPHRIC) study was performed[68]. This was a randomized, double-blind, prospective, multicenter study in 129 subjects with diabetes mellitus and serum creatinine concentrations of 1.5 to 3.5 mg/dl who were undergoing coronary or aortofemoral angiography. In the iohexol group, 17 out of 65 patients (26%) experienced a serum creatinine increase of 0.5 mg/dl or more, compared with 2 out of 64 patients in the iodixanol group (3%), with an odds ratio of 0.09 (CI 0.02–0.41, *P* = 0.002) for protection from harm with iodixanol. No patient in the iodixanol group had an increase in serum creatinine of 1.0 mg/dl or more, compared to 10 patients (15%) in the iohexol group (Figure 8.3).

Recommendations

Although complications of contrast agent administration are rare, clinicians must evaluate the risks and benefits of contrast administration in all patients, and attempt to minimize the amount of contrast administered to any patient. Still, the clinical evidence in favor of the selective use of non-ionic dimers is too limited and results of clinical studies have not been consistent. When contrast administration is clinically indicated, use of the non-ionic monomers or dimers represents currently the safest known approach to selection of iodinated intravenous contrast agents; these agents reduce the risk of CIN as well as many other complications of contrast administration.

References

1. J. Emsley, *The Elements*, Oxford Chemistry Guides (Oxford Univ. Press, New York, NY, 1995).

2. Gries J: Chemistry of X-ray contrast agents. In: Dawson P, Cosgrove DO, Grainger RG (eds): *Textbook of Contrast Media*. Oxford: ISIS Medical Media, 1999, 15–22.

3. Dawson P, Blomley MJK. Contrast Agent Pharmacokinetics Revisited. I. Reformulation. *Acad Radiol* 1995; **3**:S261–S263.

4. Dawson P, Blomley MJK. Contrast Agent Pharmacokinetics Revisited. II. Computer aided analysis. *Acad Radiol* 1995; **3**:S264–S267.

5. Dawson P, Blomley MJK. Contrast media as extracellular fluid space markers: adaptation of the central volume theorem. *Br J Radiol* 1996; **69**:717–722.

6. Dawson P, Trewhella M, Forsling M. Vasopressin release in response to intravenously injected contrast media. *Br J Radiol* 1990; **63**:97–100.

7. Petterson G, Golman K. Contrast agents of the renal tract. In: Dawson P, Cosgrove DO, Grainger RG (eds): *Textbook of Contrast Media*. Oxford: ISIS Medical Media, 1999, 121–134.

8. Dawson P. Glomerular filtration rate determined using contrast clearance: should we all be doing it? Curr Opin Urol 1996; **6**:1039–1042.

9. Mützel W, Speck U. Pharmacokinetics and biotransformation of iohexol in the rat and the dog. Acta Radiol 1980; **362(suppl)**:87–92.

10. Dawson P. Contrast agents in patients on dialysis. Sem Dial 2002; **15**:232–236.

11. Furukawa T, Ueda J, Takahashi S, Sajaguchi K. Elimination of low-osmolality contrast media by haemodialysis. *Acta Radiol* 1996; **37**:966–971.

12. Vogt B, Ferrari P, Schonholzer C, et al. Pre-emptive haemodialysis after radiocontrast media in patients with renal insufficiency is potentially harmful. *Am J Med* 2001; **111**:692–698.

13. Dehnarts T, Keller E, Gondolf K, Schiffner T, Pavenstadt H, Schollmeyer P. Effect of haemodialysis after contrast medium administration in patients with renal insufficiency. *Nephrol Dial Transplant* 1998; **13**:358–362.

14. Morisetti A, Tirone P, Luzzani F, de Haen C. Toxicological safety assessment of iomeprol, a new X-ray contrast agent. *Euro J Radiol* 1994; **18(suppl)**:S21–31.

15. Heglund IF, Michelet AA, Blazak WF, Furuhama K, Holtz E. Preclinical pharmacokinetics and general toxicology of iodixanol. *Acta Radiol* 1995; **399(suppl)**:69–82.

16. Weber G, Vigone MC, Rapa A, Bona G, Chiumello G. Neonatal transient hypothyroidism: aetiological study. *Arch Dis Child* 1998; **79(suppl)**:F70–72.

17. Dangas GD, Monsein LH, Laureno R, et al. Transient Contrast Encephalopathy After Carotid Artery Stenting. *J Endovasc Ther* 2001; **8**:111–113.

18. Sharp S, Stone J, Beach R. Contrast agent neurotoxicity presenting as subarachnoid hemorrhage. *Neurol* 1999; **52**:1503–1505.

19. Sticherling C, Berkefeld J, Auch-Schwelk, Lanfermann H. Transient bilateral cortical blindness after coronary angiography. *Lancet* 1998; **351**:570.

20. Kermode AG, Chakera T, Mastaglia FL. Low osmolar and non-ionic x-ray contrast media and cortical blindness. *Clin Exp Neurol* 1992; **29**:272–276.

21. Younathan CM, Kaude JV, Cook MD, Shaw GS, Peterson JC. Dialysis is not indicated immediately after administration of non-ionic contrast agents in patients with end-stage renal disease treated by maintenance dialysis. *Am J Roentgenol* 1994; **163**:969–971.

22. Morcos SK, Thomsen HS, Webb JA; Contrast Media Safety Committee of the European Society of Urogenital Radiology (ESUR). Dialysis and contrast media. *Eur Radiol* 2002; **12**:3026–3030.

23. Szebeni, J. Hypersensitivity Reactions to Radiocontrast Media: The Role of Complement Activation. *Curr Allergy Asthma Rep* 2004; **4**:25–30.

24. Brockow K, Christiansen C, Kanny G, et al; ENDA; the EAACI interest group on drug hypersensitivity. Management of hypersensitivity reactions to iodinated contrast media. *Allergy* 2005; **60**:150–8.

25. Katayama H, Yamaguchi K, Kozuka T, Takashima T, Seez P, Matsuura K. Adverse reactions to ionic and nonionic contrast media. A report from the Japanese Committee on the Safety of Contrast Media. *Radiology* 1990; **175**:621–628.

26. Wolf GL, Arenson RL, Cross AP. A prospective trial of ionic vs nonionic contrast agents in routine clinical practice: Comparison of adverse effects. *Am J Roentgenol* 1989; **152**:939–944.

27. Palmer FJ. The RACR survey of intravenous contrast media reactions. Final report. *Australas Radiol* 1988; **32**:426–428.

28. Caro JJ, Trindade E, McGregor M. The risks of death and of severe nonfatal reactions with high- vs low-osmolality contrast media: a meta-analysis. *Am J Roentgenol* 1991; **156**:825–832.

29. Wolf GL, Mishkin MM, Roux SG, et al. Comparison of the rates of adverse drug reactions. Ionic contrast agents, ionic agents combined with steroids, and nonionic agents. *Invest Radiol* 1991; **26**:404–410.

30. Aspelin P, Nilsson PE, Schmid-Schonbein H, Schroder S, Simon R. Effect of four non-ionic contrast media on red blood cells in vitro. I. Morphology. *Acta Radiol Suppl* 1987; **370**:79–83.

31. Aspelin P, Nilsson PE, Schmid-Schonbein H, Schroder S, Simon R. Effect of four non-ionic contrast media on red blood cells in vitro. II. Aggregation. *Acta Radiol Suppl* 1987; **370**:85–87.

32. Aspelin P, Nilsson PE, Schmid-Schonbein H, Schroder S, Simon R. Effect of four non-ionic contrast media on red blood cells in vitro. III. Deformability. *Acta Radiol Suppl* 1987; **370**:89–91.

33. Hardeman MR, Goedhart P, Koen IY. The effect of low-osmolar ionic and non-ionic contrast media on human blood viscosity, erythrocyte morphology, and aggregation behavior. *Invest Radiol* 1991; **26**: 810–819.

34. Rao VM, Rao AK, Steiner RM, Burka ER, Grainger RG, Ballas SK. The effect of ionic and nonionic contrast media on the sickling phenomenon. *Radiol* 1982; **144**:291–3.

35. Banna M. Post-angiographic blindness in a patient with sickle cell disease. *Invest Radiol* 1992; **27**: 179–181.

36. Stockman J, Nigro M, Mishkin M, Oski F. Occlusion of large cerebral vessels in sickle-cell anemia. *New Engl J Med* 1972; **287**:846–849.

37. Darr M, Hamburger S, Koprivica B, Ellereck E. Hemolytic anemia associated with a radiopague contrast agent in a patient with hemoglobin SC disease. *South Med* 1981; **174**:1552.

38. Rao AK, Thompson R, Durlacher L, James F. Angiographic contrast agent-induced acute hemolysis in a patient with hemoglobin SC disease. *Arch Int Med* 1985; **145**:759–60.

39. Raisanen J, Shapiro B, Glazer GM, Desai S, Sisson JC. Plasma catecholamines in pheochromocytoma: effect of urographic contrast media. *Am J Roentgenol* 1984; **143**:43–6.

40. Mukherjee JJ, Peppercorn PD, Reznek RH, et al. Pheochromocytoma: effect of nonionic contrast medium in CT on circulating catecholamine levels. *Radiol* 1997; **202**:227–31.

41. van der Molen AJ, Thomsen HS, Morcos SK; Contrast Media Safety Committee of the European Society of Urogenital Radiology (ESUR). Effect of iodinated contrast media on thyroid function in adults. *Eur Radiol* 2004; **14**:902–907.

42. Hintze G, Blombach O, Fink H, Burkhardt U, Köbberling J. Risk of iodine-induced thyrotoxicosis after coronary angiography: an investigation in 788 unselected subjects. *Eur J Endocrinol* 1999; **140**:264–267.

43. Martin FIR, Tress BW, Colman PG, et al. Iodine-induced hyperthyroidism due to nonionic contrast radiography in the elderly. *Am J Med* 1993; **95**:78–82.

44. Dawson P, Howell MJ. Pharmacology of the non-ionic dimers. *Br J Radiol* 1986;59:987–991.

45. Sirken G, Raja R, Garces J, Bloom E. Contrast-induced translocational hyponatremia and hyperkalemia in advanced kidney disease. *Am J Kidney Dis* 2004; **43(suppl)**:e31–5.

46. Aronson D, Dragu RE, Nakhoul F, et al. Hyponatremia as a complication of cardiac catheterization: a prospective study. *Am J Kidney Dis* 2002; **40**:940–6.

47. Swanson DP, Chilton HM, Threll JH, editors. Pharmaceuticals in medical imaging. New York: Macmillan Publishing Company, 1990: 40–42,253–77.

48. Potier M, Lagroye I, Lakhdar B, Cambar J, Idee JM. Comparative cytotoxicity of low- and high-osmolar contrast media to human fibroblasts and rat mesangial cells in culture. *Invest Radiol* 1997; **32**:62–626.

49. Schick CS, Haller C. Comparative cytotoxicity of ionic and non-ionic radiocontrast agents on MDCK cell monolayers in vitro. *Nephrol Dial Transplant* 1999; **14**:342–347.

50. Haragsim L, Zima T. [The preventive effect of calcium-channel blockers (nifedipine, verapamil) on the tabular toxicity of radiographic contrast media (Verografin, Hexabrix)] [Article in Czech] *Cas Lek Cesk* 1993; **132**:737–742.

51. Donadio C, Tramonti G, Lucchesi A, Auner I, Bianchi C. Early glomerular effects of contrast media in rats: evaluation with a simple method. *Ren Fail* 1998; **20**:20703–706.

52. Idee JM, Santus R, Beaufils H, et al. Comparative effects of low- and high-osmolar contrast media on the renal function during early degenerative gentamicin-induced nephropathy in rats. *Am J Nephrol* 1995; **15**:66–74.

53. Niu G. [Experimental histopathological studies of renal lesions induced by high- or low-osmolality contrast media] [Article in Japanese] Nippon Ika Daigaku Zasshi 1993; **60**:390–405.

54. Lancelot E, Idee JM, Couturier V, Vazin V, Corot C. Influence of the viscosity of iodixanol on medullary and cortical blood flow in the rat kidney: a potential cause of Nephrotoxicity. *J Appl Toxicol* 1999; **19**:341–346.

55. Gabelmann A, Haberstroh J, Weyrich G. Ionic and non-ionic contrast agent-mediated endothelial injury. Quantitative analysis of cell proliferation during endothelial repair. *Acta Radiol* 2001; **42**:422–425.

56. Lancelot E, Idee JM, Lacledere C, Santus R, Corot C. Effects of two dimeric iodinated contrast media on renal medullary blood perfusion and oxygenation in dogs. *Invest Radiol* 2002; **37**:368–375.

57. Sawmiller CJ, Powell RJ, Quader M, Dudrick SJ, Sumpio BE. The differential effect of contrast agents on endothelial cell and smooth muscle cell growth in vitro. *J Vasc Surg* 1998; **27**:1128–1140.

58. Scheller B, Hennen B, Thunenkotter T, et al. Effect of X-ray contrast media on blood flow properties after coronary angiography. *Thromb Res* 1999; **96**:253–260.

59. Tschakert H, Matern-Pinzek R, Schaffeldt J. [Increase of kidney enzymes in urine after administration of contrast media: comparison of the nephrotoxicity of ionic and nonionic substances] [Article in German] *Aktuelle Radiol* 1995; **5**:152–156.

60. Barrett BJ, Carlisle EJ. Metaanalysis of the relative nephrotoxicity of high- and low-osmolality iodinated contrast media. *Radiol* 1993; **188**:171–178.

61. Hill JA, Winniford M, Cohen MB, et al. Multicenter trial of ionic versus nonionic contrast media for cardiac angiography. The Iohexol Cooperative Study. *Am J Cardiol* 1993; **72**:770–5.

62. Rudnick MR, Goldfarb S, Wexler L, et al. Nephrotoxicity of ionic and nonionic contrast media in 1196 patients: a randomized trial. The Iohexol Cooperative Study. *Kidney Int* 1995; **47**:254–61.

63. Taliercio CP, Vlietstra RE, Ilstrup DM, et al. A randomized comparison of the nephrotoxicity of iopamidol and diatrizoate in high risk patients undergoing cardiac angiography. *J Am Coll Cardiol* 1991; **17**:384–90.

64. Schwab SJ, Hlatky MA, Pieper KS, et al. Contrast nephrotoxicity: a randomized controlled trial of a nonionic and an ionic radiographic contrast agent. *N Engl J Med* 1989; **320**:149–53.

65. Chalmers N, Jackson RW. Comparison of iodixanol and iohexol in renal impairment. *Br J Radiol* 1999; **72**:701–3.

66. Carraro M, Matalan F, Antonione P, et al. Effects of a dimeric vs a monomeric non-ionic contrast-medium on renal function in patients with mild to moderate renal insufficiency: a double-blind, randomized clinical trial. *Eur Radiol* 1998; **8**:144–147.

67. Kolehmainen H, Soiva M. Comparison of Xenetix 300 and Visipaque 320 in patients with renal failure. *European Radiology* 2003; **13**:B32–33.

68. Aspelin P, Aubry P, Fransson SG, Strasser R, Willenbrock R, Berg KJ. Nephrotoxicity in High-Risk Patients Study of Iso-Osmolar and Low-Osmolar Non-Ionic Contrast Media Study Investigators. Nephrotoxic effects in high-risk patients undergoing angiography. *N Engl J Med*. 2003; **348**:491–9.

120

9. PHARMACOLOGIC PROPHYLAXIS

Carlo Briguori, Flavio Airoldi, and Antonio Colombo

The mechanisms by which contrast agents induce acute renal failure are complex and not well understood. The main factors are osmotic, toxic, and hemodynamic.[1] Therefore, the optimal strategy to prevent contrast-induced nephrotoxicity remains uncertain. At present, recommendations are:

- Periprocedural hydration[2]
- Use of a low- or iso-osmolality contrast[3–6] and
- Limitation of the amount of contrast agent used[7–10]

A number of pharmacologic approaches to prevent contrast nephrotoxicity have been suggested. However, most of these strategies proved to be ineffective or harmful (Table 9.1). Recently, considerable interest has resulted from the preliminary positive data on the effectiveness of prophylactic administration of antioxidant compounds[11] and fenoldopam.[12]

Table 9.1   Pharmacologic approaches for preventing contrast-induced nephropathy

Drug	Effectivess
Vasodilators	
Atrial natriuretic peptide	No[33,34]
Calcium channel blockers	No[30]
Dopamine	No[2–35]
Endothelin antagonists	No[29]
Fenoldopam	No[12,38–40]
Antioxidants	
N-Acetylcysteine	Yes[10,11,16–24,26]
Ascorbic acid	Yes[27]
Diuretics	
Furosemide	No[2–38]
Mannitol	No[2–35]
Theophilline	Controverisal[29,35]

Antioxidant strategy

In recent years, many clinical studies have been conducted with the use of antioxidant compounds in an attempt to prevent contrast-induced nephropathy. The two most investigated drugs are acetylcysteine and ascorbic acid.

Acetylcysteine

Acetylcysteine is a potent antioxidant that scavenges a wide variety of oxygen-derived free radicals. Improvement of renal hemodynamic and prevention of direct oxidative tissue damage are among its alleged prophylactic effects against contrast-associated nephrotoxicity.[13–15] Acetylcysteine is classically known as a mucolytic agent, which is used to thin mucus, especially in patients with respiratory diseases such as emphysema, bronchitis, and cystic fibrosis. Animal experiments have shown that acetylcysteine inhibits the renal ischemia-induced reduction of c-fos and c-jun expression and the renal ischemia-induced increase of jun NH2 terminal kinase activity.[13] Tepel et al[11] firstly reported that acetylcysteine (600 mg orally twice daily) plus hydration before and after administration of contrast agent is more effective than hydration alone in preventing contrast-induced nephrotoxicity in patients with chronic renal insufficiency who were undergoing computed tomography with a constant dose (75 ml) of a non-ionic, low-osmolality contrast agent (iopromide). They prospectively studied 83 patients with chronic renal insufficiency (average serum creatinine concentration of 2.5 mg/dl [216 μmol/l]) who were randomized to either acetylcysteine (600 mg orally bid administered the day before and the day of the procedure) plus intravenous saline (0.45% at 1 ml/kg per hour for 12 hours before and 12 hours after the procedure) or to placebo plus saline. At 48 hours after administration of the contrast agent, an elevation of the serum creatinine ≥0.5 mg/dl (44 μmol/l) was much less common in the acetylcysteine group (2% versus 21%, $P=0.01$). Gastrointestinal discomfort and dizziness, the only adverse effects found, were reported in both randomized groups. Other studies eventually confirmed[16–18] and refuted[10,19,20] this preliminary observation. Due in part to these discrepant findings, the overall prophylactic efficacy of acetylcysteine has been assessed in multiple meta-analyses.[21–24] Birck et al reported a primary analysis performed among eight randomized controlled trials that enrolled 885 patients.[21] Compared with hydration alone, acetylcysteine plus hydration significantly reduced the risk of developing nephropathy after contrast administration among patients with chronic renal insufficiency (RR: 0.41; 95% CI 0.22–0.79). However, this overall effect must be viewed in the context of the marked variability in individual risk.

In a prospective study[10] that enrolled 183 patients with renal insufficiency (who had elective coronary and/or peripheral angiography, and/or angioplasty), we did not find any significant effect of acetylcysteine administration (according to the dosage suggested by Tepel et al[11]) on the occurrence of contrast-induced nephropathy. An increase of ≥25% in the baseline creatinine 48 hours after the procedure occurred in 10 out of 91 (11%) patients in the control group and in 6 out of 92 (6.5%) patients in the acetylcysteine group ($P=0.22$) (Figure 9.1, panel a). In this study the mean contrast dose was 194±127 ml (range 50–900). In the subgroup with low (<140 ml) contrast dose, renal function deterioration occurred in 5 out of 60 (8.5%) cases in the control group, and in none of 60 patients in the acetylcysteine group ($P=0.020$; OR=0.44; 95% CI=0.35–0.54). In the subgroup with high (≥140 ml) contrast dose, no difference was found

(5/31 vs 6/32, $P=0.78$) (Figure 9.1, panel b). We postulated that the discordance between our study and the previous ones[11,16–18] may be due to the amount of contrast administered. In patients undergoing coronary procedures, often requiring a large amount of contrast agent, a higher dose of acetylcysteine could be more effective than the standard dose.

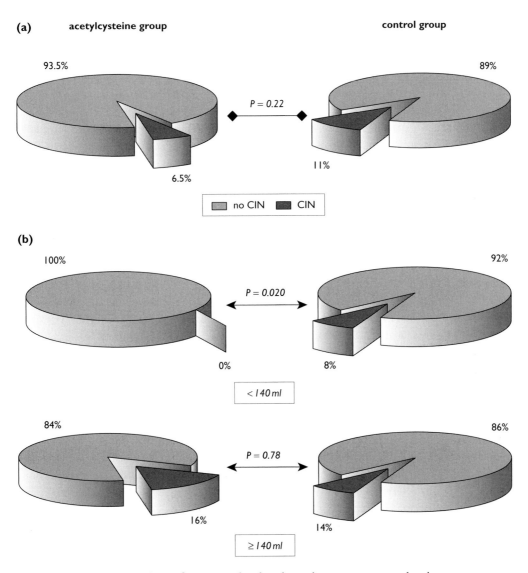

Figure 9.1 *Panel a: incidence of contrast-induced nephropathy in patients treated with N-acetylcysteine (acetylcysteine group) and in those who received hydration alone (control group). Panel b: incidence of contrast-induced nephropathy in patients who received a small (<140 ml) or a large (≥140 ml) amount of contrast dye and were treated with N-acetylcysteine (acetylcysteine group) or hydration alone (control group). CIN: contrast-induced nephropathy. (From Briguori et al.[26]).*

123

A potential mechanism of N-acetylcysteine in preventing contrast nephrotoxicity is the prevention of direct oxidative tissue damage by scavenging reactive oxygen species; this anti-oxidant effect seems to be dose-dependent. Efrati et al[25] demonstrated that treatment with N-acetylcysteine results in an increase in nitric oxide production as compared to the decrease observed in the control group after contrast agent administration. Renal vasoconstriction, possi-bly mediated by alterations in nitric oxide, and a direct toxic effect of contrast media have been implicated in the pathogenesis of contrast-induced nephrotoxicity. Contrast agents can cause a direct tubular injury, leading to the generation of oxygen free radicals, which in turn react with nitric oxide to produce peroxynitrite. Peroxynitrite is a potent oxidant that further decreases nitric oxide bioavailability and results in more tissue injury.

We therefore hypothesized that with a higher amount of contrast a higher dose of N-acetylcysteine might be necessary. In order to validate this theory, we performed a prospective, ran-domized trial in patients with baseline creatinine level ≥ 1.5 mg/dl, referred for coronary proce-dures.[26] All the 223 patients enrolled were treated with 0.45% saline intravenously according to Solomon's protocol.[2] N-Acetylcysteine was randomly administered at the standard dose (600 mg orally twice daily; SD group) or at a double dose (1200 mg orally twice daily; DD group) before and after a non-ionic, low-osmolality contrast agent administration. The median serum creatinine concentration for all patients was 1.60 (IQR=1.47–1.80) mg/dl. In the SD group, the creatinine concentration decreased from a median value of 1.56 (IQR=1.47–1.74) to 1.50 (interquartile range [IQR]=1.33–1.69) mg/dl 48 hours after contrast administration ($P=0.046$). In the DD group, the creatinine concentration decreased from a median value of 1.61 (IQR=1.45–1.86) to 1.46 (IQR=1.31–1.83) mg/dl 48 hours after contrast administration ($P<0.001$). There was a sig-nificant difference in the serum log-creatinine concentration 48 hours after contrast media admin-istration between the two treatment strategies even when including the baseline serum log-creatinine level and the amount of contrast media as covariate ($F=6.52$, $P=0.001$ by ANCOVA test). Contrast-associated nephrotoxicity (that is, an increase ≥ 0.5 mg/dl of creatinine concentra-tion) occurred in 12 out of 109 (11%) patients in the SD group and in 4 out of 114 (3.5%) patients in the DD group ($P=0.038$; OR=0.29; 95% CI=0.09–0.94) (Figure 9.2, panel a). The amount of contrast administered was higher in the 16 patients who experienced an acute contrast-associ-ated nephrotoxicity than in the remaining 207 patients (287 ± 130 ml vs. 171 ± 110 ml, $P<0.001$). Two cut-offs for high volume of contrast media were considered: (a) an absolute contrast amount of ≥ 140 ml,[10] and (b) the weight- and creatinine-adjusted maximum contrast dose (MCD=$5\times$kg body weight divided by serum creatinine [mg/dl]).[9] For each patient, the 'contrast ratio' was cal-culated as a dichotomous variable (≤ 1 or >1) dividing the amount of contrast received by the cal-culated MCD. The MCD was defined as exceeded if the contrast ratio was >1.[9] According to the selected cut-off, a large amount of contrast (≥ 140 ml) was used in 53/109 (49%) cases of the SD group and in 56/114 (49%) cases of the DD group ($P=1.0$); a contrast ratio >1 was present in 26/109 (24%) cases of the SD group and in 28/114 (25%) cases of the DD group ($P=0.88$). In patients ($n=114$) who received a contrast dose <140 ml (mean value=101 ± 23 ml; range=40–130 ml; median=100 ml), a significant renal function deterioration occurred in 2/56 (3.6%) in the SD group and in 1/58 (1.7%) in the DD group ($P=0.61$) (Figure 9.2, panel b). In patients ($n=168$) with a contrast ratio ≤ 1 (mean value=132 ± 61 ml; range=40–500 ml; median=120 ml) a significant renal function deterioration occurred in 3/82 (3.7%) in the SD group and in 1/86 (1.2%) of the DD group ($P=0.36$) (Figure 9.2, panel b). In patients who

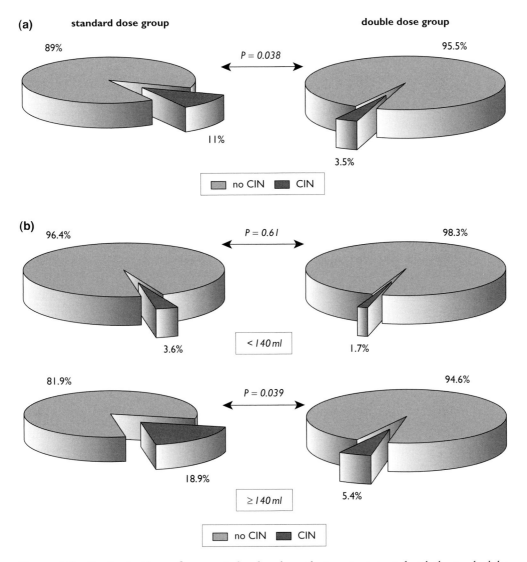

Figure 9.2 *Panel a: incidence of contrast-induced nephropathy in patients treated with the standard dose (standard dose group) or the double dose (double dose group) of acetylcysteine. Panel b: incidence of contrast-induced nephropathy in patients who received a small (< 140 ml) or a large (≥ 140 ml) amount of contrast dye and were treated with the standard dose (standard dose group) or with the double dose (double dose group) of acetylcysteine. CIN: contrast-induced nephropathy (From Briguori et al.[26]).*

received a large amount of contrast, marked deterioration of renal function occurred significantly less often in the DD group. In particular, in the subgroup ($n=109$) with contrast dose ≥ 140 ml (mean value = 254 ± 102 ml; range = 140–550 ml; median = 245 ml) this event occurred in 10/53 (18.9%) cases in the SD group, and in 3/56 (5.4%) of the DD group ($P=0.039$; OR = 0.24; 95% CI 0.06–0.94) (Figure 9.2, panel b). In the subgroup ($n=55$) with a contrast ratio > 1 (mean

125

value $= 308 \pm 111$ ml; range $= 80$–550 ml; median $= 300$ ml), a significant renal function deterioration occurred in 9/27 (31.3%) in the SD group and in 3/28 (10.7%) of the DD group ($P=0.055$; OR $=0.24$; 95% CI 0.03–1.15).

Ascorbic acid

Additional evidence of the effectiveness of the antioxidant strategy comes from the recent observations by Spargias et al, who investigated the impact of ascorbic acid in preventing contrast-induced nephrotoxicity.[27] The antioxidant ascorbic acid has been shown to attenuate renal damage in animal models caused by a variety of insults, such as postischemia stress, cisplatin, aminoglycosides, and potassium bromate, and has an extensive safety record as a dietary supplement in humans. Spargias et al conducted a randomized, double-blind, placebo-controlled trial of ascorbic acid in 231 patients with a serum creatinine concentration ≥ 1.2 mg/dl who underwent coronary angiography and/or intervention. Ascorbic acid, 3 g at least 2 hours before the procedure and 2 g in the night and the morning after the procedure, or placebo were administered orally. Hydration with 50 to 125 ml/hour iv normal saline was started in all patients from randomization until at least 6 hours after the procedure. Contrast-induced nephropathy (defined as an absolute increase of serum creatinine ≥ 0.5 mg/dl or a relative increase of $\geq 25\%$ measured 2 to 5 days after the procedure) occurred in 11 of the 118 (9%) patients in the ascorbic acid group and in 23 of the 113 (20%) patients in the placebo group (odds ratio, 0.38; 95% CI 0.17–0.85; $P=0.02$). The mean serum creatinine concentration increased significantly in the placebo group (from 1.36 ± 0.50 to 1.50 ± 0.54 mg/dl, $P<0.001$) and did not change significantly in the ascorbic acid group (from 1.46 ± 0.52 to 1.52 ± 0.64 mg/dl, $P=0.07$). The mean increase in serum creatinine concentration was greater in the placebo group than in the ascorbic acid group (difference of 0.09 mg/dl; 95% CI 0.00–0.17; $P=0.049$). In conclusion, this study supports the concept that prophylactic oral administration of ascorbic acid may protect against contrast-mediated nephropathy in high-risk patients undergoing a coronary procedure.

Inhibition of renal vasoconstriction

Due to the perturbation of renal hemodynamics induced by contrast agents, numerous vasodilator drugs have been tested for the prevention of acute reduction in renal function (Table 9.1). However, theophylline,[28,29] nifedipine,[30] and adenosine[31] do not seem to be effective. The possible importance of endothelin-induced renal vasoconstriction led to the evaluation of a non-selective endothelin receptor antagonist in a multicenter, double-blind, randomized trial of high-risk patients undergoing coronary angiography.[32] Disappointingly, a significantly higher percentage of patients who received active therapy sustained contrast nephropathy as compared with those randomized to placebo (56% vs 29%; $P=0.002$).

Atrial natriuretic peptide has been considered for prophylaxis in high-risk patients since its administration has been associated with benefits in animal models of radiocontrast-induced nephropathy.[33] However, no benefit was observed with the intravenous administration of this agent in a large multicenter, prospective, double-blind, placebo-controlled randomized trial.[34]

Although theoretically justified, studies testing the effectiveness of a low dose of dopamine showed negative or neutral results.[2–35] The failure of dopamine may be due to hypovolemia and tachyarrhythmia induced by the diuretic and pro-arrhythmogenic effects of this drug, both leading to reduced cardiac output and reduced effective circulating volume. Furthermore, the unselective stimulation of both dopamine-1 and -2 receptors may have an additional role in increasing vulnerability towards contrast-induced nephropathy.

Fenoldopam is a parenteral, selective dopaminergic agent approved in 1997 for the treatment of systemic hypertension. In contrast to dopamine, fenoldopam is a selective dopamine-1 receptor agonist with systemic and renal arteriolar vasodilator properties. This drug does not stimulate dopamine-2 or adrenergic receptors, even when administered in high doses. A low dosage of fenoldopam, that does not decrease blood pressure, produces dopamine-1 receptor-mediated and dose-related renal vasodilation, diuresis, and natriuresis when administered directly into the dog renal artery. Intravenous infusion of fenoldopam ($0.025–0.5\,\mu$/kg per min) causes small decreases in diastolic blood pressure in healthy volunteers and dose-related increases in heart rate without altering systolic blood pressure.[36] Fenoldopam significantly increases renal blood flow and decreases renal vascular resistance without altering glomerular filtration rate. In healthy volunteers, an intravenous infusion of fenoldopam ($0.025–0.5\,\mu$/kg per min) increased renal plasma flow by 12 to 57% and decreased renal vascular resistance by 19 to 42% in a generally dose-related manner.[36] Bakris et al[37] showed that fenoldopam protects against contrast-mediated reduction in renal blood flow. Kini et al[38] found that fenoldopam has a protective effect against renal ischemic injury during percutaneous coronary intervention. Intravenous fenoldopam should be started at least 1 hour before the procedure at a rate of $0.1\,\mu$g/kg per min and continued during the percutaneous intervention and for 4–6 hours after the procedure if the patient's blood pressure is stable. In the study by Kini et al,[38] that enrolled 269 patients with baseline creatinine concentration ≥ 1.5 mg/dl (mean $= 2.08 \pm 0.71$), an increase $\geq 25\%$ in creatinine level occurred in 3.8% of cases, whereas urgent dialysis was needed in 0.77%. Of note, it seems that fenoldopam extends its renoprotective benefit in patients with diabetes mellitus and baseline creatinine concentration > 2.0 mg/dl.

The evaluation of corlopam in patients at risk for renal failure (CONTRAST) was a multicenter safety and efficacy trial with a randomized, double-blind, placebo-controlled design that evaluated the effects of an iv infusion of fenoldopam in renal insufficiency patients (creatinine clearance < 60 ml/min) at risk for contrast-induced nephrotoxicity undergoing diagnostic and/or interventional procedures.[39] The CONTRAST trial showed that fenoldopam mesylate is ineffective in preventing further renal function deterioration in patients with chronic renal insufficiency receiving iodinated contrast. All 315 patients received 0.45% saline for hydration. A non-ionic contrast agent was administered to all patients and 90% of them received a low-osmolality contrast agent. Fenoldopam mesylate infusion was started at least 1 hour prior to the invasive procedure at $0.05\,\mu$g/kg per min and then increased to $0.10\,\mu$g/kg per min in 20 minutes, if tolerated. The infusion was continued during and for the 12 hours following the procedure. N-Acetylcysteine was administered prior to the procedure in 49.6% of the fenoldopam group and in 54.1% of patients in the placebo group. Premature discontinuation of the study drug due to hypotension occurred in 21% of the fenoldopam group patients compared to 11% of the patients randomized to placebo. The incidence of contrast-induced nephropathy in the fenoldopam group and in the control group was 19.9% vs 15.9% ($P=0.45$) at 48 hours, and 33.6% vs 30.1% ($P=0.61$) at

96 hours, respectively. In addition to the lack of any beneficial effect of fenoldopam, no interaction between this drug and acetylcysteine was evident.

We performed a trial in order to compare the effectiveness of fenoldopam versus acetylcysteine.[40] Patients with chronic impairment of renal function (serum creatinine concentration ≥1.5 mg/dl and/or creatinine clearance <60 ml/min) were randomly assigned to receive intravenous saline plus N-acetylcysteine (NAC group) or fenoldopam mesylate (fenoldopam group) before and after administration of iodixanol (Visipaque®, 320 mg iodine/ml, Amersham Health) a non-ionic, iso-osmolality contrast agent. Saline (0.45%) was given intravenously at a rate of 1 ml/kg of body weight per hour (0.5 ml/kg for patients with left ventricular ejection fraction [LVEF] <40%) for 12 hours before and 12 hours after administration of the contrast agent. N-Acetylcysteine (Fluimucil, Zambon Group Spa, Milan, Italy) was given orally at a dose of 1200 mg twice daily in the NAC group on the day before and on the day of administration of the contrast agent, for a total of 2 days. Fenoldopam mesylate (Corlopam, Elan Pharma, Italy) infusion was started at least 1 hour prior to contrast exposure at 0.10 μg/kg per min, maintained during the procedure and continued for 12 hours postprocedure. The dosage was reduced or discontinued in case of hypotension or tachycardia. Severe hypotension was defined as a systolic blood pressure <90 mmHg. Three patients experienced side effects in the fenoldopam group, necessitating premature drug infusion discontinuation: two patients had severe hypotension (2 and 4 hours after the procedure, respectively), and one patient had an allergic reaction (skin rush and vomiting) before the procedure. We found a trend toward a higher absolute decrease of systolic blood pressure in the fenoldopam group than in the NAC group (-17 ± 20 vs -11 ± 25 mmHg; $P=0.068$). In contrast, the decrease of diastolic (-9 ± 11 vs -9 ± 14 mmHg; $P=1.00$) and mean (-11 ± 12 vs -8 ± 15 mmHg; $P=0.30$) blood pressure was similar in the two groups. Contrast-induced nephropathy occurred in 4 out of 97(4.1%) patients in the NAC group and in 13 out of 95 (13.7%) patients in the fenoldopam group ($P=0.019$; OR=0.27; 95% CI 0.08–0.85) (Figure 9.3). Contrast-associated nephrotoxicity occurred in 5 out of 11 (45.5%) patients with a serum creatinine level >2.5 mg/dl in the fenoldopam group and in 1 out of 9 (11%) patients in the NAC

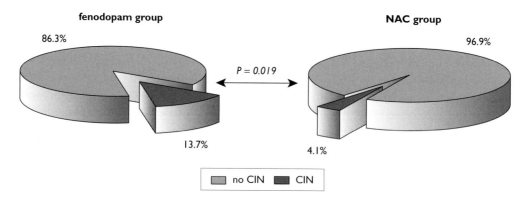

Figure 9.3 *Incidence of contrast-induced nephropathy in patients treated with fenoldopam mesylate (fenoldopam group) or N-acetylcysteine (NAC group). CIN: contrast-induced nephropathy; NAC: N-acetylcysteine. (From Briguori et al.[40]).*

group ($P=0.095$). In the 98 diabetic patients, renal function deterioration occurred in 4 out of 49 (8.2%) in the fenoldopam group and in 3 out of 49 (6.1%) in the NAC group ($P=0.72$). In the 23 patients with left ventricular ejection fraction <40%, renal function deterioration occurred in 4 out of 13 (13.3%) in the fenoldopam group and in none of the 10 in the NAC group ($P=0.23$). In patients with left ventricular ejection fraction ≥40%, renal function deterioration occurred in 9 out of 72 (12.5%) in the fenoldopam group and in 4 out of 87 (4.5%) in the NAC group ($P=0.085$). No case of contrast-associated nephrotoxicity was observed in the 16 diabetic patients with left ventricular ejection fraction <40% (7 in the fenoldopam group and 9 in the NAC group). In the fenoldopam group, mean blood pressure lowering was similar in patients with and without contrast-associated nephrotoxicity (-11 ± 11 vs -11 ± 10 mmHg; $P=0.95$), and in patients with left ventricular ejection fraction <40% and ≥40% (-13 ± 9 vs -10 ± 12 mmHg; $P=0.39$). Renal failure requiring dialysis occurred in one (1.1%) patient randomized to fenoldopam treatment; this patient subsequently died during hospitalization. Length of in-hospital stay (from admission to discharge) was longer in the fenoldopam group than NAC group (5.0 ± 10 vs 2.9 ± 2.7 days; $P=0.049$).

Based on the results of these studies, we can conclude that intravenous infusion of fenoldopam should not be used as a prophylactic measure to prevent further renal function deterioration in patients at risk for contrast-induced nephropathy.

Diuretics: mannitol and furosemide

Up to the mid-1990s, a common approach to the patient at risk for contrast nephropathy was pre-treatment with saline hydration associated with mannitol and furosemide.[2,41] However, compelling data indicate that neither mannitol nor furosemide offer additional protection against radiocontrast-induced nephrotoxicity as compared with saline hydration alone in either diabetic or non-diabetic patients.[41] In the study by Solomon et al,[2] there were no beneficial effects of the osmotic diuretic mannitol when added to saline hydration in either diabetic or non-diabetic patients, and an actual exacerbation of contrast-induced renal dysfunction was observed with the use of the loop diuretic furosemide in association with saline hydration.

The prospective randomized trial of prevention measures in patients at high risk for contrast nephropathy (PRINCE) found no benefit to force diuresis with intravenous crystalloid, furosemide, mannitol and low-dose dopamine compared to hydration alone.[41] Mannitol increases the intrarenal secretion of adenosine, a potent renal vasoconstrictor, resulting in a reduction of renal blood flow. Furthermore, the active transport process that is responsible for excretion of this osmotically active compound increases tubular mitochondrial oxygen consumption. In addition, furosemide-induced diuresis may result in hypovolemia, which may actually increase the risk of contrast-induced tubular injury.

Conclusion

Among the newer pharmacologic therapies targeted at the alleged pathophysiologic mechanisms of contrast-induced nephropathy, N-acetylcysteine and fenoldopam have been proposed as

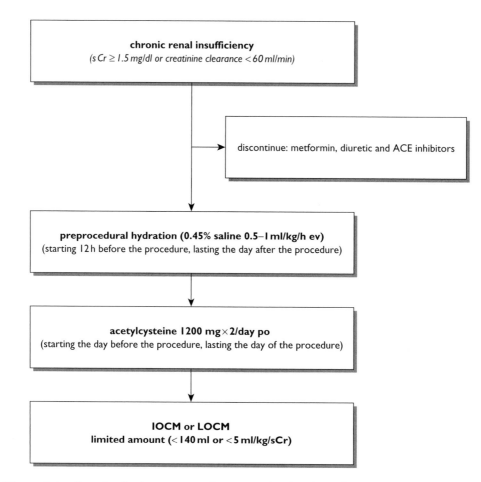

Figure 9.4 *Algorithm for the prevention of contrast-induced nephropathy in patients with chronic renal insufficiency. sCr: serum creatinine; ACE: angiotensin converting enzyme; IOCM: iso-osmolar contrast media; LOCM: low-osmolar contrast media.*

promising strategies for the prevention of this growing and serious clinical problem. Regrettably, the data from well-controlled randomized studies indicate that intravenous fenoldopam administration has no significant prophylactic effect. Moreover, the risk of hypotension and the additional cost make it an impractical approach for the prevention of contrast-associated nephropathy. However, the strategy of infusing fenoldopam directly into both renal arteries through a dedicated catheter should be further investigated (see Chapter 11). On the other hand, based on the available results, the more favorable safety profile and the low cost, acetylcysteine may be included in prophylactic protocols for patients at risk of developing contrast-induced nephropathy. In Figure 9.4 we summarize our current approach to prevent contrast-induced nephropathy in patients with pre-existing chronic renal insufficiency.

References

1. Briguori C, Tavano D, Colombo A. Contrast agent-associated nephrotoxicity. *Prog Cardiovasc Dis* 2003; **45**:493–503.

2. Solomon R, Werner C, Mann D, D'Elia J, Silva P. Effects of saline, mannitol, and furosemide on acute decreases in renal function induced by radiocontrast agents. *N Engl J Med* 1994; **331**:1416–20.

3. Rudnick MR, Goldfarb S, Wexler L et al. Nephrotoxicity of ionic and nonionic contrast media in 1196 patients: a randomized trial. *Kidney Int* 1995; **47**:254–60.

4. Schwab SJ, Hlatky MA, Pieper KS et al. Contrast nephrotoxicity: a randomized controlled trial of a nonionic and an ionic radiographic contrast agent. *N Engl J Med* 1989; **320**:149–53.

5. Barrett BJ, Carlisle EJ. Metaanalysis of the relative nephrotoxicity of high- and low-osmolality iodinated contrast media. *Radiology* 1993; **188**:171–8.

6. Steinberg EP, Moore RD, Powe NR et al. Safety and cost effectiveness of high-osmolality as compared with low-osmolality contrast material in patients undergoing cardiac angiography. *N Engl Med J* 1992; **326**:425–30.

7. Cigarroa RG, Lange RA, Williams RH, Hillis LD. Dosing of contrast material to prevent contrast nephropathy in patients with renal disease. *Am J Med* 1989; **86**:649–52.

8. McCullough PA, Wolyn R, Rocher LL et al. Acute renal failure after coronary intervention: incidence, risk factors, and relationship to mortality. *Am J Med* 1997; **103**:368–75.

9. Freeman RV, O'Donnell M, Share D et al. Nephropathy requiring dialysis after percutaneous coronary intervention and the critical role of an adjusted contrast dose. *Am J Cardiol* 2002; **90**:1068–73.

10. Briguori C, Manganelli F, Scarpato P et al. Acetylcysteine and contrast-agent associated nephrotoxicity. *J Am Coll Cardiol* 2002; **40**:298–303.

11. Tepel M, Van der Giet M, Schwarzfeld C et al. Prevention of radiographic-contrast-agent-induced reductions in renal function by acetylcysteine. *N Engl J Med* 2000; **343**:180–4.

12. Tumlip JA, Wang A, Murray PT, Mathur VS. Fenodopam mesylate blocks reduction in renal plasma flow after radiocontrast dye infusion: a pilot trial in the prevention of contrast nephropathy. *Am Heart J* 2002; **143**:894–903.

13. DiMari J, Megyesi J, Udvarhelyi N et al. N-acetylcysteine ameliorates ischemic renal failure. *Am J Physiol* 1997; **272**:F292–F298.

14. Heyman SN, Goldfarb M, Shina A, Karmeli F, Rosen S. N-acetylcysteine ameliorates renal microcirculation: studies in rats. *Kidney Int* 2003; **63**:634–41.

15. Tariq M, Morais C, Sobki A, Al Sulaiman M, Al Khader A. N-acetylcysteine attenuates cyclosporin-induced nephrotoxicity in rats. *Nephrol Dial Transplant* 1999; **14**:923–9.

16. Diaz-Sandoval LJ, Kosowsky BD, Losordo DW. Acetylcysteine to prevent angiography-related renal tissue injury (the APART trial). *Am J Cardiol* 2002; **89**:356–8.

17. Shyu KG, Cheng JJ, Kuan P. Acetylcysteine protects against acute renal damage in patients with abnormal renal function undergoing a coronary procedure. *J Am Coll Cardiol* 2002; **40**:1383–8.

18. Kay J, Chow WH, Chan TM et al. Acetylcysteine for prevention of acute deterioration of renal function following elective coronary angiography and intervention: a randomized controlled trial. *JAMA* 2003; **289**:553–8.

19. Allaqaband S, Tumuluri R, Malik AM et al. Prospective randomized study of N-acetylcysteine, fenoldopam, and saline for prevention of radiocontrast-induced nephropathy. *Cathet Cardiovasc Interven* 2002; **57**:279–83.

20. Durham JD, Caputo C, Dokko J et al. A randomized controlled trial of N-acetylcysteine to prevent contrast nephropathy in cardiac angiography. *Kidney Int* 2002; **62**:2202–7.

21. Birck R, Krzossok S, Markowetz F et al. Acetylcysteine for prevention of contrast nephropathy: meta-analysis. *Lancet* 2003; **362**:598–603.

22. Alonso A, Lau J, Jaber BL, Weintraub A, Sarnak MJ. Prevention of radiocontrast nephropathy with N-acetylcysteine in patients with chronic kidney disease: a meta-analysis of randomized, controlled trials. *Am J Kidney Dis* 2004; **43**:1–9.

23. Kshirsagar AV, Poole C, Mottl A et al. N-acetylcysteine for the prevention of radiocontrast induced nephropathy: a meta-analysis of prospective controlled trials. *J Am Soc Nephrol* 2004; **15**:761–9.

24. Pannu N, Manns B, Lee H, Tonelli M. Systematic review of the impact of N-acetylcysteine on contrast nephropathy. *Kidney Int* 2004; **65**:1366–74.

25. Efrati S, Dishy V, Averbukh M et al. The effect of N-acetylcysteine on renal function, nitric oxide, and oxidative stress after angiography. *Kidney Int* 2003; **64**:2182–7.

26. Briguori C, Colombo A, Violante A et al. Standard vs double dose of N-acetylcysteine to prevent contrast agent associated nephrotoxicity. *Eur Heart J* 2004; **25**:206–11.

27. Spargias K, Alexopoulos E, Kyrzopoulos S et al. Ascorbic acid prevents contrast-mediated nephropathy in patients with renal dysfunction undergoing coronary angiography or intervention. *Circulation* 2004; **110**:2837–42.

28. Brooks DP, DePalma PD. Blockade of radiocontrast-induced nephrotoxicity by the endothelin receptor antagonist, SB 209670. *Nephron* 1996; **72**:629–36.

29. Katholi RE, Taylor GJ, McCann WP et al. Nephrotoxicity from contrast media: attenuation with theophylline. *Radiology* 1995; **195**:17–22.

30. Bakris GL, Burnett JC Jr. A role for calcium in radiocontrast induced reduction in renal hemodynamics. *Kidney Int* 1995; **27**:465–8.

31. Pflueger A, Larson TS, Nath KA et al. Role of adenosine in contrast media-induced acute renal failure in diabetes mellitus. *Mayo Clin Proc* 2000; **75**:1275–83.

32. Wang A, Holcslaw T, Bashore TM et al. Exacerbation of radiocontrast nephrotoxicity by endothelin receptor antagonism. *Kidney Int* 2000; **57**:1675–80.

33. Margulies KB, McKinley LJ, Cavero PG, Burnett JC Jr. Induction and prevention of radiocontrast-induced nephropathy in dogs with heart failure. *Kidney Int* 1990; **38**:1101–8.

34. Kurnik BR, Allgren RL, Genter FC et al. Prospective study of atrial natriuretic peptide for the prevention of radiocontrast-induced nephropathy. *Am J Kidney Dis* 1998; **31**:674–80.

35. Abizaid A, Clark CE, Mintz GS et al. Effects of dopamine and aminophylline on contrast-induced acute renal failure after coronary angioplasty in patients with preexisting renal insufficiency. *Am J Cardiol* 1999; **83**:260–3.

36. Murphy MB, Murray C, Shorten GD. Fenoldopam: a selective peripheral dopamine-receptor agonist for the treatment of severe hypertension. *N Engl J Med* 2001; **345**:1548–57.

37. Bakris G, Lass NA, Glock D. Renal hemodynamics in radiocontrast medium-induced renal dysfunction: a role for dopamine-1 receptors. *Kidney Int* 1999; **56**:206–10.

38. Kini AS, Mitre CA, Kamran M et al. Changing trends in incidence and predictors of radiographic contrast nephropathy after percutaneous coronary intervention with use of fenoldopam. *Am J Cardiol* 2002; **89**:999–1002.

39. Stone GW, McCullough PA, Tumlin JA et al. Fenoldopam mesylate for the prevention of contrast-induced nephrotoxicity. *JAMA* 2003; **290**:2284–91.

40. Briguori C, Colombo A, Airoldi F et al. N-Acetylcysteine versus fenoldopam mesylate to prevent contrast agent-associated nephrotoxicity. *J Am Coll Cardiol* 2004; **44**:762–5.

41. Stevens MA, McCullough PA, Tobin KJ et al. A prospective randomized trial of prevention measures in patients at high risk for contrast nephropathy: results of the PRINCE study. *J Am Coll Cardiol* 1999; **33**:403–11.

10. RENAL REPLACEMENT THERAPIES

Giancarlo Marenzi and Antonio L Bartorelli

Contrast-induced nephropathy (CIN) remains an important cause of hospital-acquired acute renal failure (ARF) with major clinical and prognostic implications, particularly in patients undergoing invasive cardiovascular procedures.[1,2] Chronic renal failure (CRF), especially diabetic nephropathy, and the amount of contrast medium are considered major risk factors involved in its development. The risk of CIN increases in parallel with the decline in baseline renal function. In patients with severe CRF, defined as a creatinine clearance (CrCl) lower than 30 ml/min, the incidence of this complication increases progressively from 30% to 90–100%, whereas that of ARF, requiring temporary treatment with hemodialysis, may rise from 5% to 70–80% (Figure 10.1).[2,3] When CIN leading to dialysis occurs, a very poor clinical outcome is frequently observed, including an in-hospital mortality as high as 36% and a 2-year survival of only 19%.[4,5]

The nephrotoxic effect of contrast medium is dose-dependent: the higher the volume of contrast used, the higher the risk. However, more than the absolute contrast volume, the interaction of contrast volume and renal function is the key factor determining the risk of CIN.[6] As the glomerular filtration rate (GFR) declines, a lesser amount of contrast is enough to induce this serious and potentially fatal complication. In patients with severely depressed GFR (< 30 ml/min),

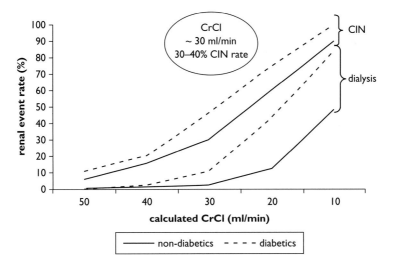

Figure 10.1 *Validated risk of contrast-induced nephropathy (CIN) and acute renal failure requiring dialysis after diagnostic angiography and ad-hoc angioplasty in non-diabetic and diabetic patients. A mean contrast dose of 250 ml and a mean age of 65 is assumed. CrCl: creatinine clearance; CIN: contrast-induced nephropathy.*

even 15 to 30 ml of contrast can cause ARF, leading to dialysis.[7] Registry and trial data have shown that the average dose of contrast used for coronary angiography is 130 ml, and for percutaneous coronary interventions (PCI) is 191 ml.[8,9] Thus, despite the fact that different strategies are being advocated which would minimize the amount of contrast administered, invasive coronary procedures represent a very serious hazard in patients with impaired renal function.

CIN is usually predictable, due to the fact that its risk factors are well known. This offers an opportunity to utilize preventive strategies. Among several prophylactic approaches, only hydration and the use of antioxidant agents (acetylcysteine, ascorbic acid), bicarbonate, and iso-osmolar and low-osmolar contrast agents have been shown to provide some protection.[10–15] However, their efficacy in patients with severe CRF is still controversial, and their impact on clinical outcome is completely unknown. To date, patients with severe CRF, undergoing coronary angiography and PCI, continue to have a risk of CIN that approximates 50%, and an associated cardiovascular death rate of 30% within 1 year.[16–18] In endstage renal disease, chronic dialysis treatment does not offer significant protection against this increased risk. In two studies, the 2-year survival of dialysis patients after PCI was reported to range between 48% and 53%.[19,20]

Hence, more effective prophylactic strategies are needed to attenuate the particularly high risk associated with invasive cardiovascular procedures in patients with CRF. The potential protective effects and therapeutic advantage of a non-pharmacologic approach, based on the use of renal replacement therapies (RRT), such as hemodialysis, hemofiltration, and hemodiafiltration, have been a matter of intense investigative interest in recent years.

Rationale for the use of RRT to prevent and treat CIN

The pharmacokinetic properties of contrast media are such that they are distributed in the extracellular fluid only, are minimally bound to circulating proteins, are not metabolized, and are mainly excreted by glomerular filtration. When renal function is normal, the half-life of contrast agents is approximately 2 hours, but it can be prolonged to over 30 hours in patients with severe CRF, in proportion to the extent of renal impairment.[21] Contrast media may remain in extracellular body fluids for several days in patients with severe renal failure.[22] If toxicity of contrast media on tubular cells is one of the pathophysiologic mechanisms leading to CIN, removal of contrast media may be of clinical benefit. Effective contrast removal by the artificial membranes used with RRT, through a process similar to spontaneous glomerular filtration, has been demonstrated in CRF patients. Plasma levels of several different contrast media are reported to be reduced by 60–80% with hemodialysis.[23] By contributing to residual endogenous clearance, this may reduce the risk of CIN. Schindler et al[24] compared, in a randomized study, the ability of different dialysis modalities to remove contrast media in patients on chronic dialysis treatment and in those with CRF (serum creatinine [Cr] >4 mg/dl) not yet on RRT. They demonstrated that different RRT modalities, started with a mean interval of 1.2 ± 0.6 hours from the radiologic procedure, effectively removed contrast media. However, the highest contrast clearance (114 ± 4 ml/min) was observed for hemodiafiltration, a procedure that combines convective and diffusive solute removal, followed by high-flux hemodialysis (100 ± 2.2 ml/min), hemofiltration (86 ± 5 ml/min), and low-flux hemodialysis (82 ± 2.3 ml/min). The elimination of dye from the circulation by RRT

Table 10.1 Factors that influence the elimination of contrast media by hemodialysis

Contrast media
  Molecular size and weight
  Protein binding
  Electrical charge
  Hydrophilicity

Hemodialysis procedure
  Permeability and surface area of the filter membrane
  Membrane material
  Blood flow rate
  Dialysate flow rate
  Duration of procedure

Patient factors
  Degree of hepatic and renal excretion
  Contrast medium plasma concentration

can be influenced by several factors (Table 10.1). They include: (a) intrinsic characteristics of the contrast media molecules such as size and weight (the smaller the solute molecule, the more easily it moves across the membranes), plasma protein binding (the higher the hydrophilicity, as in non-ionic contrast media, the lower the protein affinity), and electrical charge; (b) degree of residual renal excretion in non-anuric patients, and (c) extracorporeal treatment characteristics including membrane surface area, blood and dialysate flow rates, and treatment duration.[21] Peritoneal dialysis is also effective in removing contrast agents from the body but it requires a longer time than hemodialysis.[25]

Prevention of CIN with RRT

Hemodialysis

On the basis of studies demonstrating its effectiveness in contrast media removal, hemodialysis (HD) (Figure 10.2) has been proposed as a CIN preventive strategy after radiographic procedures. However, no definitive benefit on the incidence of CIN and clinical outcome has been demonstrated in randomized trials (Table 10.2). The first clinical study with HD was carried out by Moon et al[26] in 20 CRF patients who were on chronic HD treatment ($n = 7$) or not ($n = 13$). HD was started with a delay of 1 to 18 hours after angiographic procedures, and was continued for 6 hours. No increase in Cr was reported in these patients. However, the study design did not include a control group, so the HD prophylactic effect remains uncertain. Two subsequent studies, involving relatively small populations, failed to confirm a positive effect of HD. In the study of Lehnert et al,[17] 30 patients with CRF (mean Cr 2.4 mg/dl) were randomized in order to receive either an intravenous infusion of isotonic saline (83 ml/hour), for 12 hours before contrast agent exposure

135

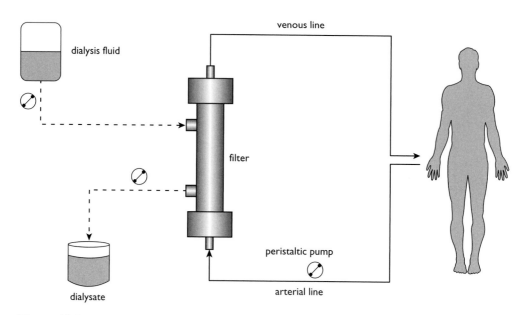

Figure 10.2 *Graphic representation of the extracorporeal circuit used in hemodialysis.*

(3 ml/kg body weight), followed by HD (dialysate flow of 500 ml/min without fluid withdrawal) for 3 hours, started as soon as possible after contrast injection (mean delay 63 ± 6 minutes), or an intravenous hydration, administered for 12 hours before and 12 hours after the radiographic procedure. The incidence of CIN in the HD group and in the control group was 53% and 40%, respectively. Thus, no clear benefit of HD over hydration was demonstrated, despite confirmation of an effective extracorporeal plasma clearance achieved by HD. The same results were obtained by Sterner et al[27] in 32 patients with CRF, randomized into a single HD treatment or a standard treatment after angiography. This study again confirmed the ability of hemodialysis to decrease the plasmatic concentration of contrast (iohexol) and the lack of a CIN preventive effect.

More recently, in a large randomized clinical study performed by Vogt et al,[28] prophylactic HD in the prevention of CIN was evaluated in 113 patients with CRF (Cr > 2.3 mg/dl). Of these, 58 patients were assigned to receive saline intravenous infusion (1 ml/kg per hour) for 12 hours, before and after administration of the contrast agent, and 55 to receive saline infusion before contrast media exposure, followed by HD that was started between 30 and 280 minutes (median 120 minutes) after contrast media injection. HD was continued for about 3 hours with a dialysate flow of 500 ml/min and without net ultrafiltration in most patients. The baseline Cr value was similar in the two groups (3.5 and 3.6 mg/dl, respectively), whereas the mean dose of contrast was higher in the HD group (200 ± 19 ml vs 143 ± 15 ml; $P = 0.007$). In addition, a higher proportion of HD group patients underwent coronary angiography (45% vs 22%; $P = 0.006$). A similar incidence of CIN was observed in the two groups (16% in the control group and 24% in the hemodialysis group; $P = 0.35$). Similarly, there was no significant difference in major in-hospital events (stroke, pulmonary edema, myocardial infarction, and death). Finally, a greater percentage of patients treated with HD required additional HD treatment, or had declines in renal function,

Table 10.2 Randomized studies evaluating hemodialysis for the prevention of contrast-induced nephropathy

Reference	Patients (n)	Baseline renal function	Treatment duration	Contrast agent	Dose of contrast agent	CIN incidence
Lehnert et al[17]	30	2.58 ± 0.25 mg/dl / 2.26 ± 0.2 mg/dl	3 hours	Iopentol	3.5 ± 0.6 ml/kg / 3.0 ± 0.4 ml/kg	53% / 40% / P=NS
Sterner et al[27]	32	3.6 mg/dl / 3.0 mg/dl	4 hours	Iohexol (n=13) Iodixanol (n=11) Ioxaglat (n=8)	17 g iodine / 17 g iodine	NA / NA
Vogt et al[28]	113	3.5 ± 1.2 mg/dl / 3.6 ± 1.3 mg/dl	3.1 ± 0.7 hours	LOCM	210 ± 143 ml / 143 ± 115 ml	24% / 16% / P=NS
Frank et al[33]	17	3.9 ± 1.3 mg/dl / 4.2 ± 1.1 mg/dl	4 hours	Iomeprol	77.3 ± 27.4 ml / 85.6 ± 21.2 ml	28% / 20% / P=NS

For each study, the values in *italic* refer to control groups.
CIN: contrast-induced nephropathy; LOCM: low-osmolality contrast medium; NA: not available.

137

than did those treated with saline hydration alone. The authors concluded that prophylactic HD after contrast media exposure was not beneficial, and even potentially harmful. The lack of benefit observed with HD in this study may be due, at least in part, to the different amount of dye administered in the two groups, and to the fact that coronary angiography was performed twice as often in the HD group, raising the possibility that these patients were exposed to a higher risk.

In summary, all these studies show that the strategy of performing HD immediately after administration of contrast media in patients with reduced renal function does not prevent CIN. The incongruence between the effective removal of contrast media by HD and the lack of a preventive effect against CIN may be the result of HD-related nephrotoxicity, caused by activation of inflammatory reactions, coagulation processes, and release of vasoactive substances that may induce acute hypotension.[29] Furthermore, hemodynamic instability due to the osmotic shift of fluid from the intravascular to the interstitial and intracellular compartments, and to the dialysis-associated ultra-filtration, is frequently observed during HD.[30,31] Hypovolemia can induce renal hypoperfusion, vasoconstriction, and ischemic injury. Thus, the hemodynamic consequences of HD may offset the positive effect deriving from the removal of contrast agent from the circulation. A third possible reason may be the rapid onset of renal injury, after administration of contrast media, that may occur before starting HD. Renal hypoperfusion has been noted within 20 minutes after the injection of contrast media, suggesting that the renal injury may occur at its first renal passage.[32] In most of the studies, contrast removal by HD was started after a relatively long time, even hours, after the initial injection of the agent. Thus, the explanation for the lack of clinical benefit could be that the delay between exposure to and elimination of the contrast agents was too long.

In an attempt to obviate to this issue, Frank et al[33] investigated the effect of HD performed during contrast media administration. In this study, 17 patients with CRF (Cr ≥ 3 mg/dl) received preprocedure hydration with 1000 ml of 0.9% saline solution over a time period of 6 hours, and were randomly assigned to high-flux HD, started 10 minutes before angiography and continued for 4 hours (n = 7), or to continuous intravenous hydration for 6 hours (n = 10). Plasma levels of radiocontrast material (iomeprol) were measured at several time points. Consistent with previous findings, clearance of iomeprol was significantly greater (54 ± 15 ml/min) in the group that underwent HD when compared with the control group (20 ± 12 ml/min; $P < 0.001$). However, the incidence of CIN was similar (28% vs 20%, respectively). Of note, plasma peak levels of iomeprol were detected 15 minutes after coronary angiography, and did not significantly differ between the two groups. The peak value of dye concentration, more than the time to which kidneys are exposed to it, is thought to be the major pharmacokinetic factor responsible for CIN. Indeed, several experimental studies have shown that renal vasoconstriction following contrast agent exposure is initiated by the first renal passage, and caused by the release of mediators such as endothelin-1, which has been shown to depend on peak plasma concentrations of the contrast agent.[32,34,35] In conclusion, the hypothesis that a simultaneous HD therapy may protect the patient from CIN could not be demonstrated, presumably because plasma peak concentration of the contrast agent was not affected by this type of RRT.

Hemodiafiltration

Hemodiafiltration (Figure 10.3) offers potential advantages in comparison to HD in terms of contrast agent extracorporeal clearance efficacy and of greater hemodynamic stability.

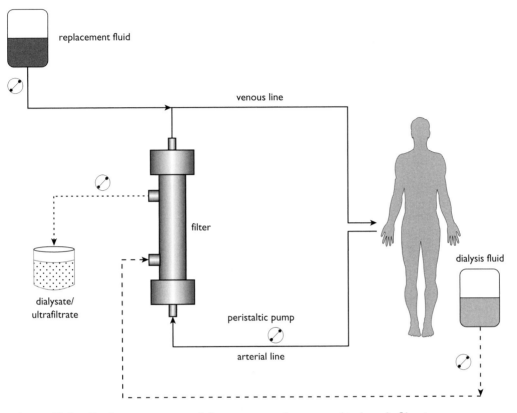

Figure 10.3 Graphic representation of the extracorporeal circuit used in hemodiafiltration.

Hemodiafiltration is a dialytic procedure that is hemodynamically and metabolically better tolerated than HD.[36] Gabutti et al[37] investigated the feasibility and efficacy of continuous venovenous hemodiafiltration, performed during and after invasive cardiovascular procedures, mainly coronary and peripheral angiographies, in preventing CIN in 26 patients with multiple risk factors: CRF (mean CrCl of 29 ml/min; $n = 22$), diabetic nephropathy ($n = 11$), and hypovolemia and/or low cardiac output ($n = 8$). Hemodiafiltration was started immediately before the contrast agent administration, and was continued for about 10 hours at a blood flow rate of 150 ml/min and a dialysis and replacement fluid flow rate of 2 l/hour (both solutions containing bicarbonate as buffer). The incidence of CIN was compared with a historic control group ($n = 25$) with mild to severe CRF. The procedure was hemodynamically well tolerated in all cases. CIN occurred in 37% of treated patients and 24% of the historic control group, indicating that even this type of RRT does not offer any appreciable protection against contrast-induced nephrotoxicity.

Hemofiltration

In contrast to these results, a recent study from our Institute provided evidence that hemofiltration (HF) (Figure 10.4), a simpler form of RRT, offers protection against CIN in high-risk

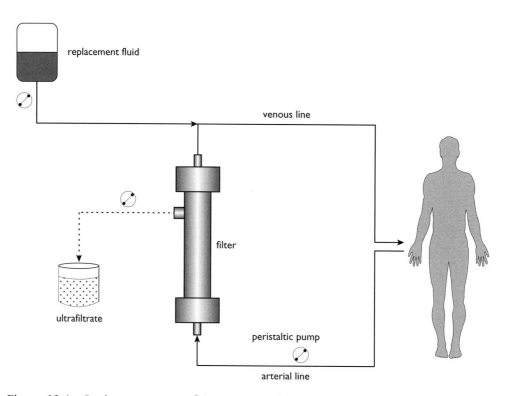

Figure 10.4   *Graphic representation of the extracorporeal circuit used in hemofiltration.*

patients.[16] One hundred and fourteen consecutive patients with advanced CRF undergoing PCI were randomly assigned to either HF ($n = 58$, mean Cr value 3.0 ± 1.0 mg/dl) or isotonic saline hydration ($n = 56$, mean Cr value 3.1 ± 1.0 mg/dl, infusion rate 1 ml/kg per hour). Treatment was initiated 4 to 6 hours before radiocontrast administration, stopped for the duration of the angiographic procedure, and resumed and continued for 18 to 24 hours after the procedure. HF was performed in an intensive care unit, using a double-lumen catheter inserted in a femoral vein; the fluid replacement rate was set at 1000 ml/hour without weight loss. CIN developed in only 3 of 58 (5%) patients in the HF group, and in 28 of 56 (50%) patients in the control group ($P < 0.001$). The study also evaluated the rate of in-hospital and long-term (12-month follow-up) outcomes (Figure 10.5 and Table 10.3). No patient in the HF group required emergency HD, whereas 10 of 56 (18%) patients in the control group needed HD. There was only 1 (2%) death in the HF group compared with 8 (14%) deaths in the control group ($P = 0.02$). The cumulative 1-year mortality was 10% and 30% for the HF and control groups, respectively ($P = 0.01$). In the control group, the relative risk of death within 1 year was 1.16 among patients with a baseline Cr level less than 4 mg/dl (95% CI 0.96–1.40; $P = 0.11$), and 3.53 (95% CI 1.08–1.20; $P = 0.002$) among patients with a baseline Cr level of 4 mg/dl or greater when compared with the HF group. This study demonstrated that prophylactic HF protects patients with advanced CRF against the development of CIN. Moreover, it was the first clinical study to show that reduction of CIN rate positively impacts in-hospital and long-term outcomes in patients known to be at considerable

140

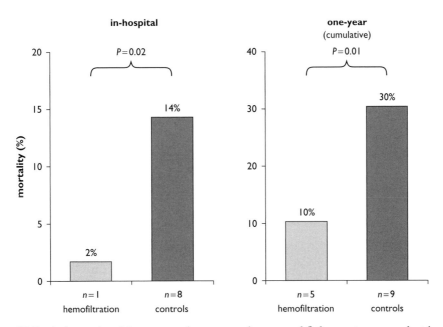

Figure 10.5 *In-hospital and 1-year mortality rates in chronic renal failure patients treated with hemofiltration and in controls.*

Table 10.3 Postprocedural complications of patients with advanced chronic renal failure (mean creatinine 3.1 ± 1.0 mg/dl) undergoing PCI with or without hemofiltration preventive treatment

	Hemofiltration group (n = 58)	Control group (n = 56)	P value
Q-wave MI	0 (0%)	2 (4%)	NS
Non-Q-wave MI	1 (2%)	1 (2%)	NS
Emergency CABG	0 (0%)	0 (0%)	NS
Pulmonary edema	0 (0%)	6 (11%)	0.02
Hypotension/shock	1 (2%)	3 (5%)	NS
Blood transfusion	1 (2%)	3 (5%)	NS
RRT	2 (3%)	14 (25%)	<0.001
All clinical events	5 (9%)	29 (52%)	<0.001

CABG: coronary artery bypass graft surgery; MI: myocardial infarction; PCI: percutaneous coronary intervention; RRT: renal replacement therapy (hemodialysis, hemofiltration).

risk. The findings are particularly noteworthy because the beneficial effects of hemofiltration, that were greater than all previous prophylactic strategies tested, were evident, despite the large amount of contrast medium administered (mean dose about 250 ml).

The mechanisms involved in the prophylactic effect of HF remain unclear. Positive effects may derive from its ability to remove contrast agent from the circulation, thereby reducing kidney exposure to its nephrotoxic effects. However, despite the fact that this action has been demonstrated,[24] it is unlikely that it plays a major role, given the negative results obtained with HD and hemodiafiltration, two more efficient forms of solute removal. Thus, other mechanisms are likely to be implicated. The most important difference between this and the other previous investigations with RRT is that HF was started 4 to 6 hours before contrast agent administration. This suggests that pre-PCI treatment may be a major factor for the preventive renal effect of this technique. This hypothesis is strongly supported by the results of a recent randomized clinical study, in which two different HF protocols for the prevention of CIN were compared.[38] In this study, 92 consecutive patients with severe CRF (CrCl < 30 ml/min), scheduled for elective cardiovascular procedures, were randomized in order to receive one of the following three prophylactic treatments: intravenous hydration with isotonic saline, performed for 12 hours before and for 12 hours after contrast exposure (control group, $n = 30$, mean Cr 3.6 ± 0.8 mg/dl), intravenous hydration with isotonic saline, performed for 12 hours before contrast exposure, followed by HF treatment for 18 to 24 hours after the procedure (post-HF group, $n = 31$; Cr 3.6 ± 0.7 mg/dl), and HF performed for 6 hours before and for 18 to 24 hours after contrast exposure (pre/post-HF group, $n = 31$; Cr 3.7 ± 0.9 mg/dl). Risk factors for CIN in addition to CRF were present in most patients.

Twelve (40%) patients of the control group experienced CIN, as compared with 8 (26%) of the post-HF group, whereas only 1 patient (3%) of the pre/post-HF group developed this renal complication ($P = 0.0013$) (Figure 10.6). Emergency HD or HF for CIN-related ARF was required in 9 (30%) control patients, in 3 (10%) post-HF patients, and in none of the pre/post-HF group ($P = 0.002$). Nine (10%) patients died during the hospitalization period for cardiovascular causes: 6 (20%) in the control group, 3 (10%) in the post-HF group, and none (0%) in the pre/post-HF group ($P = 0.03$) (Table 10.4). This study confirms that prophylactic HF is particularly effective in preventing CIN and the associated poor outcome in high-risk patients. In addition, these results may help to clarify some of the mechanism(s) involved in its beneficial effect. The marked reduction of the CIN preventive effect when only post-HF was performed indicates that a preprocedural session is necessarily required in order to obtain the full clinical benefit of HF. This may explain the results of the previous studies in which prophylactic RRT, started during or at different times after the administration of contrast media, did not result in any significant reduction in the degree of

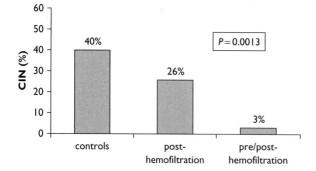

Figure 10.6 *Incidence of contrast-induced nephropathy (CIN) in controls, in patients treated with hemofiltration only after contrast medium administration (post-hemofiltration), and in patients treated with hemofiltration before and after contrast medium administration (pre/post-hemofiltration). (From Marenzi et al.[38]).*

Table 10.4 Postprocedural complications in patients with severe chronic renal failure (CrCl < 30 ml/min) undergoing PCI and randomized to hydration alone, hydration and hemofiltration after contrast medium administration, or hydration and hemofiltration performed before and after contrast medium administration

	Controls (n = 30)	Post-hemofiltration (n = 31)	Pre/Post-hemofiltration (n = 31)	P value
Acute myocardial infarction	5 (17%)	4 (13%)	1 (3%)	0.21
Emergency CABG	0 (0%)	0 (0%)	0 (0%)	—
Pulmonary edema requiring MV	1 (3%)	1 (3%)	0 (0%)	0.59
Cardiogenic shock requiring IABP	1 (3%)	0 (0%)	0 (0%)	0.35
Blood transfusion	4 (13%)	6 (19%)	5 (16%)	0.81
ARF requiring RRT	9 (30%)	3 (10%)	0 (0%)	0.002
≥2 clinical complications	6 (20%)	2 (6%)	0 (0%)	0.019
Contrast-induced nephropathy	12 (40%)	8 (26%)	1 (3%)	0.0013
In-hospital mortality	6 (20%)	3 (10%)	0 (0%)	0.02

ARF: acute renal failure; CABG: coronary artery bypass graft surgery; CMA: contrast medium administration; IABP: intra-aortic balloon pump; MV: mechanical ventilation; PCI: percutaneous coronary intervention; RRT: renal replacement therapy (hemodialysis, hemofiltration).
From Marenzi et al[38].

renal injury when compared to saline hydration alone.[17,24,26–28,33] On the other hand, the need for a preprocedural session of HF suggests that controlled high-volume hydration plays a major role in kidney protection from the contrast- agent-induced toxic injury. Hydration with saline solution still represents the 'gold standard' of CIN prophylaxis.[10,11] However, vigorous hydration before contrast exposure CMA is difficult logistically, and is poorly tolerated, in particular in the presence of impaired cardiac and renal function. A substantial fluid administration and the consequent intravascular volume expansion without a parallel fluid removal increase the risk of vascular congestion and pulmonary edema.

When patients are treated with HF, the replacement fluid infusion in the outflow loop of the circuit is comparable to intravenous hydration, with the relevant advantage that infusion rate can be markedly increased (from 10 to 15 times with the protocol utilized in these studies). Moreover, fluid elimination is precisely controlled by ultrafiltration so that hypervolemia and extravascular fluid accumulation are prevented. It can also be speculated that, in addition to high-volume controlled hydration, removal of mediators of contrast-induced toxicity by convective filtration and adsorption to the filter membrane may play a significant role.[34,39] Finally, an adjunctive renoprotective effect could also derive from the alkalizing bicarbonate-based solutions that are used as replacement fluid during HF.[14] Thus, vigorous hydration with high-volume alkaline solutions could markedly amplify the benefits obtained with simple intravenous hydration, without the risk of vascular congestion and pulmonary edema.

Treatment of CIN-induced ARF by RRT

Intermittent HD continues to be the preferred treatment of CIN-related ARF. However, no clear evidence of its superiority over other kinds of RRT has ever been demonstrated. In particular, a form of RRT, simpler than HD, such as HF, permits effective fluid and solute removal with greater fluid volume control, and, from the logistic standpoint, without requiring the availability of trained dialysis personnel. Moreover, HF offers better cardiovascular stability in critically ill patients than does conventional intermittent HD, and this represents a clear advantage, especially in the treatment of ARF in patients with associated cardiac insufficiency.[40,41] Until now, controlled studies have not shown a definite advantage of HF, in comparison with HD, in patient survival.[42-45] Furthermore, the selection of the best RRT modality may differ in different clinical situations, and no comparative studies have ever been performed in order to investigate the possible superiority of HF over HD in ARF complicating procedural cardiovascular procedures.

In our institute, we evaluated the clinical results of HF obtained in 33 patients who developed CIN-related oligo-anuric ARF after PCI, with ($n = 20$) or without ($n = 13$) associated overt congestive heart failure.[46] Treatment with HF was continued for 4.7 ± 2.6 days, and was associated with a recovery of spontaneous diuresis, improvement in renal function parameters, and correction of fluid and electrolyte imbalance in all but one patient. Notably, HF was associated with cardiovascular stability, even in those patients in whom several liters of fluid had been withdrawn. All patients were at high risk for CIN, due to the presence of pre-existing CRF (67%), diabetes (48%), reduced left ventricular function (55%), and congestive heart failure (45%). Furthermore, in 13 patients (39%), PCI was complicated by critical hemodynamic instability due to ventricular fibrillation ($n = 1$), acute pulmonary edema ($n = 4$), cardiogenic shock ($n = 2$), severe bleeding ($n = 2$), and prolonged systemic hypotension ($n = 4$). In this complex population, in-hospital mortality rate was 9.1% ($n = 3$). In all but one of the surviving patients, diuresis recovered, and HF could be terminated. Six patients died during the 12-month follow-up, accounting for a cumulative 1-year mortality of 27.3%.

This is the first clinical experience with HF in this particular clinical setting, and, thus, larger and randomized studies comparing HF with standard HD are required to fully assess the clinical benefit of this alternative form of RRT in patients developing ARF after PCI. It is, however, noteworthy that the mortality rate of this study population was significantly lower than that reported for historic controls who were treated with intermittent HD (Figure 10.7). Gruberg et al[47] reported an in-hospital and 1-year mortality of 27.5% and 54.5%, respectively, in 51 patients requiring HD treatment after percutaneous coronary interventions. An in-hospital mortality of 35% and a 2-year survival of 19% were reported by McCullough et al.[4] In another study of Gruberg et al,[48] in-hospital mortality of patients requiring HD was 22.6%, whereas the cumulative 1-year mortality was 45%. The remarkably lower in-hospital and 1-year mortality of HF-treated patients (9% and 27%, respectively) suggest a potential clinical advantage of this technique over HD in patients suffering ARF after contrast exposure. This could be related to the greater hemodynamic stability offered by HF that only rarely is complicated by hypovolemia and hypotension.[41] Hypotension and hemodynamic instability during RRT may worsen renal

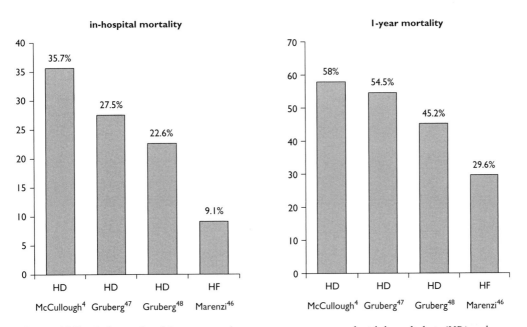

Figure 10.7 *In-hospital and 1-year mortality rates in patients treated with hemodialysis (HD) and hemofiltration (HF) for acute renal failure due to contrast-induced nephropathy.*

ischemic injury, delay ARF recovery, and prolong treatment duration.[49,50] These prerogatives seem to be confirmed by some retrospective studies showing a trend toward shorter anuria and treatment duration in patients undergoing HF, as compared with those treated by intermittent HD, although little is known about the influence of the two procedures on the duration of ARF.[51,52]

Conclusions

In conclusion, the interest in using an RRT for the prevention of CIN in high-risk patients has not vanished, but has only progressively moved from a postprocedural to a preprocedural application (Figure 10.8), and focused on the possibility of obtaining a safe and hemodynamically tolerated high-volume hydration, rather than a mechanical removal of contrast agent. Hemofiltration represents an important advance in CIN prevention, because it is the first strategy to effectively attenuate the risk of CIN, allowing us to extend the range of patients with advanced CRF who can undergo invasive cardiovascular procedures safely. Further investigation, however, is needed to confirm the positive clinical impact of such an approach, to better elucidate the mechanisms through which HF exerts its positive effects, and to identify patients and clinical settings in which the greatest benefit can be obtained.

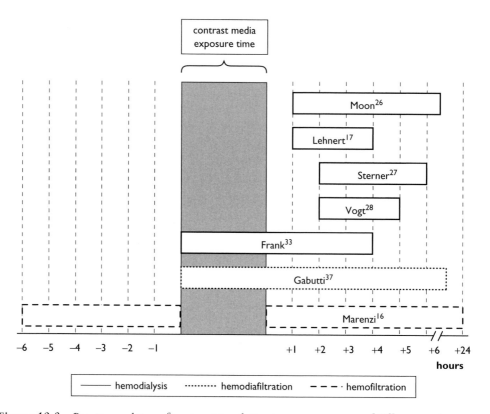

Figure 10.8 *Duration and time of treatment in relation to contrast exposure of different renal replacement therapies used in clinical studies.*

References

1. Gleeson TG, Bulugahapitiya S. Contrast-induced nephropathy. *AJR* 2004; **183**:1673–89.
2. Rihal CS, Textor SC, Grill DE et al. Incidence and prognostic importance of acute renal failure after percutaneous coronary intervention. *Circulation* 2002; **105**:2259–64.
3. McCullough PA, Sandberg KR. Epidemiology of contrast-induced nephropathy. *Rev Cardiovasc Med* 2003; **4**:S3–S9.
4. McCullough PA, Wolyn R, Rocher LL, Levin RN, O'Neill WW. Acute renal failure after coronary intervention: incidence, risk factors and relationship to mortality. *Am J Med* 1997; **103**:368–75.
5. Gruber L, Mehran R, Dangas G et al. Acute renal failure requiring dialysis after percutaneous coronary interventions. *Cathet Cardiovasc Interven* 2001; **52**:409–16.
6. Cigarroa RG, Lange RA, Williams RH, Hillis LD. Dosing of contrast material to prevent contrast nephropathy in patients with renal disease. *Am J Med* 1989; **86**:649–52.
7. Manske CL, Sprafka JM, Strony JT. Contrast nephropathy in azotemic diabetic patients undergoing coronary angiography. *Am J Med* 1990; **89**:615–20.
8. Noto TJ, Johnson LE, Krone R et al. Cardiac catheterization 1990: a report of the registry of the Society for Cardiac Angiography and Interventions. *Cathet Cardiovasc Diagn* 1991; **24**:75–83.
9. Davidson CJ, Laskey WK, Hermiller JB et al. Randomized trial of contrast-media utilization in high-risk PTCA. The COURT trial. *Circulation* 2000; **101**:2172–7.

10. Solomon R, Werner C, Mann D, D'Ella J, Silva P. Effects of saline, mannitol, and furosemide on acute changes in renal function induced by radiocontrast agents. *N Engl J Med* 1994; **331**:403–11.

11. Mueller C, Buerkle G, Buettner HJ et al. Prevention of contrast media-associated nephropathy: randomized comparison of 2 hydration regimens in 1620 patients undergoing coronary angioplasty. *Arch Intern Med* 2002; **162**:329–36.

12. Briguori C, Manganelli F, Scarpato P et al. Acetylcysteine and contrast agent-associated nephrotoxicity. *J Am Coll Cardiol* 2002; **40**:298–303.

13. Spargias K, Alexopoulos E, Kyrzopoulos S et al. Ascorbic acid prevents contrast-mediated nephropathy in patients with renal dysfunction undergoing coronary angiography or intervention. *Circulation* 2004; **110**:2837–42.

14. Merten GJ, Burgess WP, Gray LV et al. Prevention of contrast-induced nephropathy with sodium bicarbonate. A randomized controlled trial. *J Am Med Assoc* 2004; **291**:2328–34.

15. Aspelin P, Aubry P, Fransson SG et al. Nephrotoxic effects in high-risk patients undergoing angiography. A double-blind randomized multicenter study of iso-osmolar and low-osmolar non-ionic contrast media. *N Engl J Med* 2003; **348**:491–9.

16. Marenzi G, Marana I, Lauri G et al. The prevention of radiocontrast-agent-induced nephropathy by hemofiltration. *N Engl J Med* 2003; **349**:1331–8.

17. Lehnert T, Keller E, Gondolf K et al. Effect of hemodialysis after contrast medium administration in patients with renal insufficiency. *Nephrol Dial Transplant* 1998; **13**:358–62.

18. Hemmelgarn BR, Ghali WA, Quan HQ et al. Poor long-term survival after coronary angiography in patients with renal insufficiency. *Am J Kidney Dis* 2001; **37**:64–72.

19. Herzog CA, Ma JZ, Collins AJ. Long-term outcome of dialysis patients in the United States with coronary revascularization procedures. *Kidney Int* 1999; **56**:324–32.

20. Herzog CA, Ma JZ, Collins AJ. Comparative survival of dialysis patients in the United States after coronary angioplasty, coronary artery stenting, and coronary artery bypass surgery and impact of diabetes. *Circulation* 2002; **106**:2207–11.

21. Morcos SK, Thomsen HS, Webb JAW et al. Dialysis and contrast media. *Eur Radiol* 2002; **12**:3026–30.

22. Nossen JO, Jakobsen JA, Kjaersgaard P et al. Elimination of the non-ionic X-ray contrast media iodixanol and iohexol in patients with severely impaired renal function. *Scand J Clin Lab Invest* 1995; **55**:341–50.

23. Waaler A, Svaland M, Fauchald P et al. Elimination of iohexol, a low-osmolar nonionic contrast medium, by hemodialysis in patients with chronic renal failure. *Nephron* 1990; **56**:871–5.

24. Schindler R, Stahl C, Venz S et al. Removal of contrast media by different extracorporeal treatments. *Nephrol Dial Transplant* 2001; **16**:1471–4.

25. Brooks MH, Barry KG. Removal of iodinated contrast material by peritoneal dialysis. *Nephron* 1973; **12**:10–14.

26. Moon SS, Back SE, Kurkus J, Nilsson-Ehle P. Hemodialysis for elimination of the nonionic contrast medium iohexol after angiography in patients with impaired renal function. *Nephron* 1995; **70**:430–7.

27. Sterner G, Frennby B, Kurkus J et al. Does post-angiographic hemodialysis reduce the risk of contrast medium nephropathy? *Scand J Urol Nephrol* 2000; **34**:323–6.

28. Vogt B, Ferrari P, Schonholzer C et al. Prophylactic hemodialysis after radiocontrast media in patients with renal insufficiency is potentially harmful. *Am J Med* 2001; **111**:692–8.

29. Herbelin A, Nguyen AT, Zingraff J, Urena P, Descamps-Latscha B. Influence of uremia and hemodialysis on circulating interleukin-1 and tumor necrosis factor alpha. *Kidney Int* 1990; **37**:116–25.

30. Collins AJ, Keshaviah P, Ilstrup KM, Shapiro F. Clinical comparison of hemodialysis and hemofiltration. *Kidney Int* 1985; **17**:S18–S22.

31. Santoro A, Mancini E, Zucchelli P. The impact of hemofiltration on the systemic cardiovascular response. *Nephrol Dial Transplant* 2000; **15**:49–54.

32. Russo D, Minutolo R, Cianciaruso B et al. Early effects of contrast media on renal hemodynamics and tubular function in chronic renal failure. *Am J Soc Nephrol* 1995; **6**:1451–8.

33. Frank H, Werner D, Lorusso V et al. Simultaneous hemodialysis during coronary angiography fails to prevent radiocontrast-induced nephropathy in chronic renal failure. *Clin Nephrol* 2003; **60**:176–82.

34. Cantley LG, Spokes K, Clark B et al. Role of endothelin and prostaglandins in radiocontrast-induced renal artery constriction. *Kidney Int* 1993; **44**:1217–23.

35. Tublin MF, Murphy ME, Tessler FN. Current concepts in contrast media-induced nephropathy. *AJR* 1998; **171**:933–9.

36. Maggiore Q, Pizzarelli F, Dattolo P, Maggiore U, Cerrai T. Cardiovascular stability during haemodialysis, haemofiltration and haemodiafiltration. *Nephrol Dial Transplant* 2000; **15**:68–73.

37. Gabutti L, Marone C, Monti M et al. Does continuous venovenous hemodiafiltration concomitant with radiological procedures provide a significant and safe removal of the iodinated contrast ioversol? *Blood Purif* 2003; **21**:152–7.

38. Marenzi G, Lauri G, Campodonico J et al. Comparison of two hemofiltration protocols for prevention of contrast-induced nephropathy in high-risk patients. *Am J Med* 2006. In press.

39. Heyman SN, Rosen S. Dye-induced nephropathy. *Semin Nephrol* 2003; **23**:477–85.

40. Bellomo R, Ronco C. Continuous renal replacement therapy in the intensive care unit. *Int Care Med* 1999; **25**:781–9.

41. Marenzi G, Lauri G, Grazi M et al. Circulatory response to fluid overload removal by extracorporeal ultrafiltration in refractory congestive heart failure. *J Am Coll Cardiol* 2001; **38**:963–8.

42. Kellum Ja, Metha RL, Angus DC et al. The first international consensus conference on continuous renal replacement therapy. *Kidney Int* 2002; **62**:1855–63.

43. Metha RL, McDonald B, Gabbai FB et al. Collaborative Group for Treatment of ARF in the ICU. A randomized clinical trial of continuous versus intermittent dialysis for acute renal failure. *Kidney Int* 2001; **60**:1154–63.

44. Tonelli M, Manns B, Feller-Kopman D. Acute renal failure in the intensive care unit: a systematic review of the impact of dialytic modalities on mortality and renal recovery. *Am J Kidney Dis* 2002; **40**:875–85.

45. Teehan GS, Liangos O, Lau J et al. Dialysis membrane and modalità in acute renal failure: understanding discordant meta-analysis. *Semin Dial* 2003; **16**:356–60.

46. Marenzi G, Bartorelli AL, Lauri G et al. Continuous veno-venous hemofiltration for the treatment of contrast-induced acute renal failure after percutaneous coronary interventions. *Cathet Cardiovasc Interven* 2003; **58**:59–64.

47. Gruber L, Mehran R, Dangas G et al. Acute renal failure requiring dialysis after percutaneous coronary interventions. *Cathet Cardiovasc Interven* 2001; **52**:409–16.

48. Gruberg L, Mintz GS, Mehran R et al. The prognostic implications of further renal function deterioration within 48 hours of interventional coronary procedures in patients with pre-existent chronic renal insufficiency. *J Am Coll Cardiol* 2000; **36**:1542–8.

49. Murray P, Hall J. Renal replacement therapy for acute renal failure. *Am J Respir Crit Care Med* 2000; **162**:777–81.

50. Paganini EP, O'Hara P, Nakomoto S. Slow continuous ultrafiltration in hemodialysis-resistant oliguric acute renal failure patients. *ASAIO Trans* 1984; **30**:173–7.

51. van Bommel EFH. Are continuous therapies superior to intermittent hemodialysis in the acute renal failure on the intensive care unit? *Nephrol Dial Transplant* 1995; **10**:311–14.

52. Kierdorf HP, Sieberth HG. Continuous renal replacement therapies versus intermittent hemodialysis in acute renal failure: what do we know? *Am J Kidney Dis* 1996; **28**:S90–S96.

11. NOVEL PREVENTIVE STRATEGIES FOR CONTRAST-INDUCED NEPHROPATHY

Vandana S Mathur

Targeted renal delivery

Failed drug strategies for contrast-induced nephropathy – an issue of local dose?

There are no proven therapeutic pharmacologic agents for the prevention or treatment of acute renal failure generally or for contrast-induced nephropathy specifically. Although a number of drugs have been studied, including several vasodilators (Table 11.1), none has been successful via systemic administration. It is known, however, for many drugs that the optimal renal response requires drug doses that are higher than those that are systemically tolerable. This 'kidney–body disconnect' may be a particularly important issue in patients with acute and chronic renal insufficiency who often have resistance to the renal actions of drugs intended to elicit effects on the kidneys. Accumulating evidence suggests that targeted renal delivery of drugs with favorable renal effects leads both to enhanced renal effects and reduced systemic exposure and systemic effect, such that the therapeutic window for renal drugs may be enhanced by this route of delivery. The application of targeted renal therapy in the prevention of contrast nephropathy is discussed.

Medullary hypoxia as the dominant mechanism of contrast-induced nephropathy

Oxygen diffuses from the descending to ascending vasa recta in the mammalian kidney, effectively 'short-circuiting' oxygen delivery to the renal medulla. In fact, under normal conditions, the

Table 11.1 Systemically administered renal vasodilators shown to be ineffective for prevention of contrast-induced nephropathy	
Drug or drug class	Reference
Dopamine	Weisberg et al 1994[1]
Fenoldopam	Stone et al 2003[2]
Atrial natriuretic peptide	Kurnik et al 1990[3]
Mixed endothelin antagonists	Wang et al 2000[4]
Nifedipine	Khoury et al 1995[5]

medulla of mammalian kidneys functions at pO_2 as low as 30 mmHg. Both high-osmolar as well as non-ionic and low-osmolar radiocontrast agents reduce renal papillary blood flow such that red blood cell movement is greatly diminished and red cells aggregate. As a result, radiocontrast administration causes oxygen tension within the medulla to fall substantially.[6,7] Moreover, contrast agents redistribute renal blood flow such that blood flow from the vulnerable medulla is shunted to the relatively well-perfused renal cortex.[8]

The short supply of oxygen in the renal medulla is aggravated by high metabolic demand related to the work of electrolyte transport.[8] A number of mechanisms are operational in normal kidneys, including nitric oxide and vasodilator prostaglandins that prevent acute tubular necrosis.[9] However, under conditions in which one or more protective factors are diminished (i.e. during use of non-steroidal anti-inflammatory drugs), renal ischemia can develop following exposure to radiocontrast agents.[10,11] Indeed, clinical risk factors for contrast nephropathy are conditions in which medullary oxygenation may be impaired. In patients with chronic kidney disease, remnant nephrons are hyper-trophied and have structurally altered medullary microcirculation.[8] Additionally risk factors such as volume depletion, nephrotic syndrome, heart failure, and cirrhosis are all associated with reduced effective circulation, which, in turn, may adversely affect medullary oxygenation (Figure 11.1).

Although a direct tubular toxic injury from radiocontrast agents is conceivable as another factor in the pathogenesis of contrast-induced nephropathy, several observations argue against an important role of direct tubular toxicity:[8]

- Although histologic tubular vacuolar changes and simplification of the brush border can be observed, these changes have no correlation with renal dysfunction.[11–13]
- The ability of the kidneys to reabsorb sodium remains intact.
- Urinary levels of KIM-1 (kidney ischemia molecule), a marker of tubular injury, are not increased in patients with clinical contrast-induced nephropathy.[14]

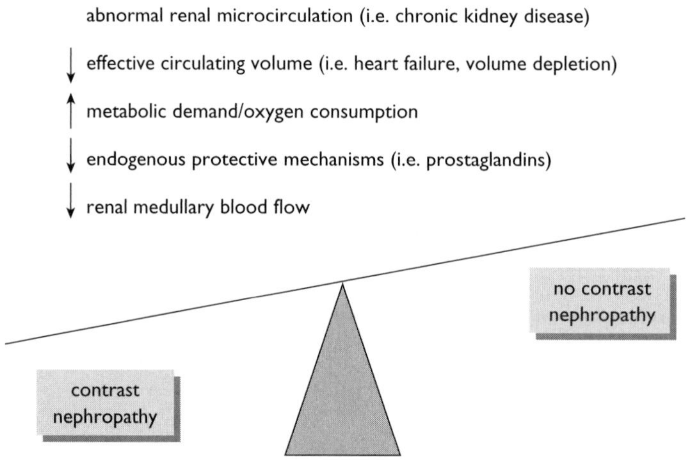

abnormal renal microcirculation (i.e. chronic kidney disease)

↓ effective circulating volume (i.e. heart failure, volume depletion)

↑ metabolic demand/oxygen consumption

↓ endogenous protective mechanisms (i.e. prostaglandins)

↓ renal medullary blood flow

no contrast nephropathy

contrast nephropathy

Figure 11.1 *Pathophysiologic factors contributing to renal medullary hypoxemia and the development of contrast-induced nephropathy.*

150

As the aggravation of medullary hypoxemia is central to the pathogenesis of contrast-induced nephropathy, drugs that increase blood flow to the kidney either directly or indirectly by reducing local or circulating renal vasoconstrictors and those that reduce metabolic demand within the kidneys are potential therapeutic candidates. Amongst renal vasodilators, those drugs that preferentially enhance medullary circulation are most likely to be effective at preventing or treating contrast-induced nephropathy.

Targeted renal therapy

The concept of targeting delivery of drugs with desirable renal effects is based on several premises:

- Infusion of drugs that are metabolized or excreted by the kidneys will, due to 'renal-first-pass' elimination, allow the delivery of therapeutically relevant or optimal renal doses of drugs to the kidneys while limiting systemic exposure.
- Targeted delivery of drugs will have greater renal effects due to higher local concentrations.
- Neurohormonally mediated renal vasoconstriction may be decreased by suppression of the renin–angiotensin–aldosterone axis and production of adrenal norepinephrine.

Because the perfusion to the adrenal gland is, in part, by an arterial branch off the main renal artery, infusion of drugs with neurohormonal suppressive properties (i.e. natriuretic peptides) into the renal vasculature may be more effective when given via the intrarenal (IR) route (Figure 11.2).

In the context of interventional cardiology, targeted renal therapy may be performed during the index diagnostic or interventional procedures with currently available systems (see below).

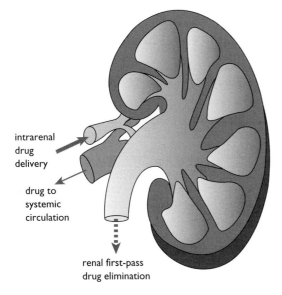

intrarenal drug delivery

drug to systemic circulation

renal first-pass drug elimination

Figure 11.2 *Targeted renal therapy. Targeted renal therapy is a strategy of improving the therapeutic window for drugs with beneficial renal effects. Drug is delivered directly into the renal arteries such that high renal and adrenal concentrations may be achieved. Due to renal first-pass elimination, the majority of drug is excreted into the urine and only a minority is available to return to the systemic circulation via the renal vein. Therefore, systemic drug exposure and adverse events related to the drug are minimized.*

Systems for targeted renal therapy

Until recently, there was no practical means by which to simultaneously and selectively deliver drugs into both kidneys. However, systems that enable bilateral renal drug delivery both within the context of angiography and in other situations have been recently commercialized.

The Ben*ephit*™ Infusion System (FlowMedica, Inc., Fremont, CA, United States) was the first commercially available device in both the United States and Europe to enable targeted renal therapy. Designed to allow bilateral renal infusion during a coronary or peripheral angiography procedure, the device consists of a selective radio-opaque bifurcated infusion catheter (Figures 11.3 and 11.4) and an 8 Fr introducer sheath (Figure 11.3). The system is indicated for the infusion of physician-specified agents into the peripheral vasculature, including the renal arteries. The bifurcated infusion catheter is an agent delivery device, which contains a 77 cm (working length) infusion lumen,

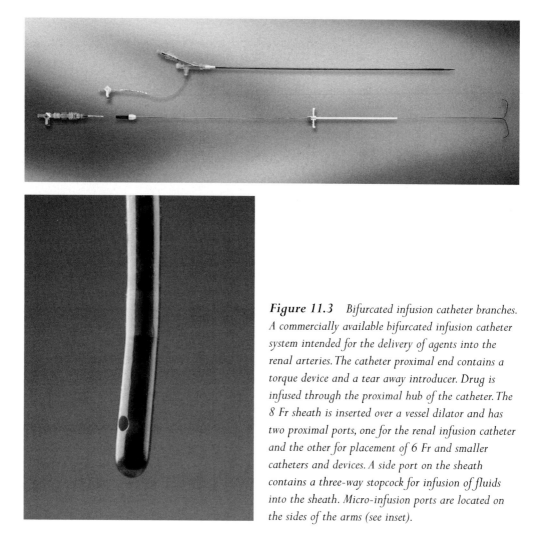

Figure 11.3 *Bifurcated infusion catheter branches. A commercially available bifurcated infusion catheter system intended for the delivery of agents into the renal arteries. The catheter proximal end contains a torque device and a tear away introducer. Drug is infused through the proximal hub of the catheter. The 8 Fr sheath is inserted over a vessel dilator and has two proximal ports, one for the renal infusion catheter and the other for placement of 6 Fr and smaller catheters and devices. A side port on the sheath contains a three-way stopcock for infusion of fluids into the sheath. Micro-infusion ports are located on the sides of the arms (see inset).*

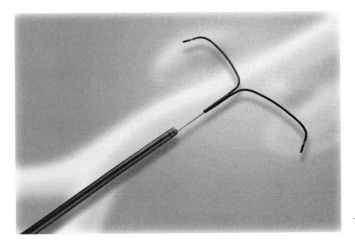

Figure 11.4 Benephit^{TM} infusion catheter arms. The radio-opaque tips are atraumatic and the 3.1 Fr branches are very flexible to accommodate renal artery anatomic variations.

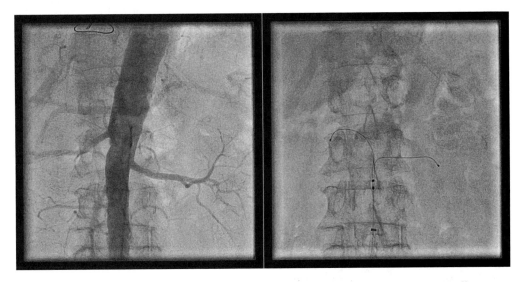

Figure 11.5 (Left) An aortic 'roadmap' image depicting renal arteries with a large vertical offset. (Right) Bilateral renal cannulation with the Benephit Infusion System in the same patient.

bifurcated at the distal end into two identical 3.1 Fr infusion branches. These are designed to allow rapid and selective cannulation of the renal arteries bilaterally without the need for guide wires. Once placed, simultaneous bilateral drug infusion may be performed. The bifurcated infusion catheter is designed for use with the system's introducer sheath. The introducer sheath (which is available in four lengths) provides for the introduction of the Benephit^{TM} System Catheter to the renal arteries and the introduction of the standard coronary (or peripheral) guiding or diagnostic catheters (6 Fr and smaller) through a second port for the diagnostic angiography or interventional procedure. Use of the Benephit^{TM} System Sheath, therefore, allows both renal drug infusion and coronary or peripheral angiography to be performed simultaneously using only a single arterial access site. The flexible branches of the catheter accommodate a wide range of renal anatomic variations, including large offsets between renal arteries (Figure 11.5); this facilitates bilateral cannulation that, in clinical studies, was accomplished in the vast majority within seconds or minutes (see below).

Systems are also available for patients who may benefit from targeted renal therapy for ischemic renal conditions in non-angiography clinical settings (i.e. heart failure with cardiorenal syndrome, hepatorenal syndrome, and intra- and postsurgical acute tubular necrosis). The Be*nephit*™ Delta Infusion System (FlowMedica, Inc., Fremont, CA, United States), for example, allows delivery, through a 5 Fr sheath, of a bifurcated renal infusion catheter that has been specifically developed to accommodate longer infusion durations and alternative entry sites (radial artery, brachial artery) in addition to the femoral approach.

Drug candidates for targeted renal therapy

Agents with vasodilator, anticonstrictive, or cytoprotective effects are potential candidates for targeted renal therapy for kidney protection. Drugs that are eliminated or metabolized by the kidneys, but that have systemic side-effects, would be particularly well suited to this route of delivery as renal efficacy of the drug could be enhanced while systemic effect is diminished. A partial list of agents or drug classes that meet such criteria is given in Table 11.2.

Several agents (fenoldopam, B-type natriuretic peptide (nesiritide), sodium bicarbonate, and a Iprostadil) are already being investigated for delivery via the IR route for prevention of contrast-induced nephropathy. The above agents can favorably affect renal physiology and are eliminated by the kidneys. Additionally, both nesiritide and fenoldopam have dose-related renal effects; however, for both, doses that elicit robust renal effects also produce hypotension.[15–17] Systemic administration of large volumes of sodium bicarbonate are limited by the risk of pulmonary edema in patients with impaired ventricular function and system alkalosis.

Fenoldopam: a case study drug for targeted renal therapy

Fenoldopam, a dopamine (DA)-1 specific receptor agonist, serves as an excellent example of a promising renoprotective drug that has been difficult to administer in renal therapeutic doses due to dose-related systemic hypotension. However, with administration, the desirable renal effects are enhanced and systemic exposure and blood pressure reduction significantly decreases.

The pharmacologic actions of fenoldopam include dose-dependent renal and systemic arterial vasodilation and natriuresis and diuresis.[16,28] Unlike dopamine, fenoldopam has no agonist action on α- or β-adrenergic receptors at any dose. Fenoldopam is currently marketed in the United States and parts of Europe and Asia for the indication of intravenous treatment of hypertension.

Studies of intravenous fenoldopam

The mechanism of action of fenoldopam is well suited for prevention of contrast-induced nephropathy – it increases blood flow (and therefore oxygen delivery) to the renal medulla,[29] which is most vulnerable to renal ischemia, and it also may reduce renal metabolic demand by inhibiting sodium reabsorption.[30] In animal models, fenoldopam attenuates reduction of glomerular filtration rate (GFR) and renal blood flow in animal models of radiocontrast nephropathy.[31] However, because the doses of fenoldopam that produce systemic vasodilation[32] overlap with the

Table 11.2 Potential agents or drug classes for intrarenal delivery for contrast nephropathy prevention

Agent or drug class	Desired renal effect	Undesirable systemic effect
Dopamine receptor agonists[16,18] Fenoldopam Dopexamine Dopamine	Direct renal vasodilation Increase renal medullary blood flow Inhibit sodium reabsorption Maintain glomerular filtration rate	Hypotension (fenoldopam, dopexamine) Hypertension, renal and systemic vasoconstriction, arrhythmias (dopamine)
Natriuretic peptides[19–21] Atrial natriuretic peptide B-type natriuretic peptide Dendroaspis natriuretic peptide Urodilatin	Anticonstriction of renal vasculature Inhibit sodium reabsorption	Hypotension
Adenosine antagonists[22]	Maintain glomerular filtration rate	Hypotension
Endothelin type A receptor antagonists[8,23]	Increase medullary blood flow	Hypotension
Prostaglandin E₁ analogues[24]	Anticonstriction of renal vasculature	Hypotension
Vasopressin antagonists[8]	Increase medullary blood flow	Unknown
High-volume sodium chloride[25]	Dilute and reduce viscosity of tubular fluid Reduce tubular debris Increase medullary blood flow	Volume overload
Sodium bicarbonate[26]	Decrease oxidation stress	Volume overload, alkalosis
N-Acetylcysteine[27]	Scavenge free radicals	None identified

doses that produce renal vasodilation,[16] optimal renal dosing of fenoldopam via systemic infusion may not be generally achievable.

Several initial studies, mostly conducted using titration protocols aimed at increasing fenoldopam to high doses ($0.5\,\mu g/kg$ per min), suggested that this agent was effective at preventing radiocontrast nephropathy in high-risk patients (serum creatinine $\geq 1.5\,mg/dl$).[33,34] However, subsequent randomized trials performed using lower doses ($0.05–0.1\,\mu g/kg$ per min) noted that these doses did not increase glomerular filtration rate[17] or prevent contrast-induced nephropathy in patients with chronic kidney disease.[35] The fact that approximately 25% of patients in the largest trial (CONTRAST)[35] could not be titrated even to the low (target) dose of 0.1 µg/kg per min suggests that choosing higher drug doses for the trial may not, in fact, have been feasible.

Studies of intrarenal fenoldopam

To determine whether targeting the kidneys with fenoldopam would, due to 'renal-first-pass', limit systemic exposure and allow the delivery of optimal renal doses, fenoldopam was infused directly into both renal arteries for 6 hours using the Benephit™ Infusion System in a series of crossover-design canine pharmacokinetic experiments. It was demonstrated that systemic fenoldopam levels were higher by approximately 70–99% following intravenous (IV) delivery vs IR delivery, suggesting a substantial renal first-pass effect of fenoldopam. Furthermore, the systemic hypotensive effects during IV infusion were attenuated with IR infusion. Bilateral renal cannulation took under 3 minutes[36] and there were no gross or histologic abnormalities noted in the kidneys or vasculature. This dog model has been proven subsequently to be highly predictive of human effects of fenoldopam.

A recent multicenter, randomized, controlled trial demonstrated significant differences in systemic levels and blood pressures following IV vs IR fenoldopam treatment (using the Benephit™ Infusion System) in patients with renal insufficiency undergoing angiography procedures.[37] A single-center study of 20 patients in which fenoldopam was administered either IV or into a single renal artery during cardiac catheterization reported similar differential effects on blood pressure.[38]

Further, in the multicenter study above, it was found that the GFR (using inulin clearance) increased by 4.5% following 30 minutes of IV treatment (steady state) with fenoldopam (0.2 µg/kg per min); however, GFR increased by approximately 19% after only 5–10 minutes of IR treatment at the same dose. The GFR effects of IR, but not IV fenoldopam, were significantly better than placebo and the differences in GFR following IV vs IR fenoldopam were also significantly different. The fact that in this study IV fenoldopam doses of 0.2 µg/kg per min, a dose 2–4 times that used in the CONTRAST trial above, did not affect GFR in patients, suggests a plausible explanation for the failure of that trial.

These studies together demonstrated the feasibility, tolerability, and safety of IR fenoldopam administered through the Benephit™ Infusion System. Additionally, the data support the hypothesis that targeted renal therapy may widen the therapeutic window for renal therapeutics by allowing delivery of higher doses than would be systemically tolerable or by achieving otherwise unattainable renal effects. Further, these studies form the basis for the hypothesis that IR fenoldopam infusion will prevent contrast-induced nephropathy. A multicenter randomized controlled trial is ongoing to further evaluate IR fenoldopam infusion in diabetic patients at extremely high risk for contrast-induced nephropathy (serum creatinine ≥ 2.0 mg/dl or creatinine clearance ≤ 35 ml/min).

In addition to ongoing randomized clinical trials, data are being collected on 'real-world' usage patterns, device performance characteristics, efficacy, and safety data in the Benephit System Renal Infusion Therapy Registry (Be-RITe!). Consecutive patients who have been treated with the Benephit™ Infusion System based on clinically determined need at selected study centers are enrolled retrospectively in this observational study. The study protocol does not dictate any particular drug treatments or patient characteristics, but, rather, captures data on clinical application of the device.

The initial experience from the Be-RITe! database was recently reported.[39] Twenty-three patients were enrolled by eight interventional cardiologists at five United States institutions. Baseline, procedural, performance, drug infusion, treatment goal, and efficacy data are reported in Tables 11.3 and 11.4.

156

Table 11.3   Clinical and procedural characteristics of the Be-RITe! Registry patients

Baseline characteristics	
Age (years)	66±10
Gender (male)	87%
Serum creatinine (mg/dl)	2.3±1.2
Serum creatinine ≥2.5 mg/dl	26%
Patient factors contributing to decision to use targeted renal therapy	
Chronic kidney disease	91.3%
Diabetes mellitus	47.8%
Congestive heart failure	26.0%
Low left ventricular ejection fraction	17.3%
Anticipated use of high volume of contrast	17.3%
Acute renal failure	4.0%
Physician-specified goals for targeted renal therapy	
Increase renal perfusion	59.1%
Prevent acute renal failure	95.0%
Increase urine output	22.7%
Treat acute renal failure	4.5%
Adjunctive procedures	
Percutaneous coronary angioplasty	45.4%
Coronary stent	68.1%
Total contrast volume (ml)	200±135
Number of devices exchanged through the second port of the sheath (within a guiding catheter or directly)	4.4±3.4
Closure device used	45.4%
Intrarenal drug treatment	
Median duration of IR drug infusion (hours)	0.77
Range of duration of IR drug infusion (hours)	0.15–4.5

(Continued)

Table 11.3 *(Continued)*	
Fenoldopam starting dose (μg/kg per min)	0.19±0.06
Fenoldopam ending dose (μg/kg per min)	0.35±0.20
Systemic anticoagulation	
IV Heparin (bolus/infusion)	57%/8.7%
Bivalirudin (bolus/infusion)	26%/22%
No systemic anticoagulation	4.3%

Table 11.4 Performance and efficacy results of the Benephit™ Infusion System in the Be-RITe! Registry	
Device performance	
Device preparation problems	0%
Problems positioning the sheath	0%
Contrast volume for aortic roadmap to place device (median, ml)	10.0
Bilateral renal artery cannulation	83.0%
Unilateral renal artery cannulation	17.0%
Renal artery cannulation time (median, minutes)	2.0
Successful infusion of physician-specified drug (when attempted)	100%
Problems removing catheter	0%
Parameters of efficacy	
Clinical goals of targeted renal therapy achieved	95.0%
Creatinine decreased	27.8%
Creatinine did not increase	67.7%
Dialysis required	0%
Data are expressed as means ± SD or percentages unless otherwise specified.	

One patient received IR alprostadil (40 ng/kg per min), the rest received IR fenoldopam (0.1–0.8 μg/kg per min). Renal cannulation was successfully accomplished despite as much as a 75% renal artery stenosis and situations of acute caudal renal artery take-off. In four cases, only a single renal artery cannulation was possible due to renal artery stenosis or other anatomic difficulties. There were no device-related complications or adverse events. The catheter dislodged in three instances during device exchange, but was easily placed back into position.

The Be*nephi*t Infusion System performed very well and was safe in the hands of multiple physicians at several institutions in a cohort of patients at high risk for development of contrast nephropathy. Despite the intraprocedural discovery of a broad range of renal artery anatomic variations and significant vascular disease, bilateral renal artery cannulation was accomplished in 83% of patients in a median of 2.0 minutes. The serum creatinine decreased or did not rise postprocedure in 96.5% of patients and, despite the high-risk patient profile, no patients required dialysis.

Studies of intrarenal nesiritide

B-Type natriuretic peptide (BNP) has a number of potential useful renal effects for the prevention and treatment of acute renal failure. These include suppression of renin, norepinephrine, endothelin-1, and diuresis/natriuresis.[19] Anticonstriction of renal vasculature may lead to renal protective effects in heart failure and other renal vasoconstrictive states such as radiocontrast nephropathy.

Clearance of BNP occurs by several routes, all of which exist within the kidneys: degradation by neutral endopeptidase, receptor-mediated clearance, and by glomerular filtration. As such, it would be predicted that IR nesiritide delivery would be largely eliminated on first pass through the kidneys.

In fact, pharmacology and pharmacokinetic crossover-design studies of nesiritide in dogs have shown that systemic exposure following IV vs IR administration (via the Be*nephi*t Infusion System) was approximately 60–75% higher, suggesting a substantial renal first-pass elimination effect.[40] Correlating with the above, systemic hypotensive effects during IV infusion were attenuated with IR infusion. No gross or microscopic histopathologic injuries of the aorta, renal arteries, or kidneys were observed.

Several human trials are in progress to better define the renal effects of nesiritide in patients with acute and chronic renal insufficiency undergoing diagnostic or interventional procedures or who have heart failure.

Contrast removal

Contrast-induced nephropathy is a unique example of a form of renal failure in which the moment of exposure to the toxic insult can be fully predicted. Moreover, numerous studies suggest that dose of contrast correlates with the risk of developing contrast-induced nephropathy. Due to this, there has been interest in the use of systems that either remove contrast soon after it is given (i.e. with renal replacement therapies, which are more fully discussed in Chapter 10) or even during the procedure before it reaches the kidneys.

The latter novel approach involves a percutaneous catheter-based device to remove contrast agent directly from the coronary sinus before it reaches the kidneys. The contrast aspiration mechanism is activated when an optical sensor detects the presence of contrast.

Prototype systems for contrast aspiration are being developed to enable testing of this strategy in animal models.

References

1. Weisberg LS, Kurnik PB, Kurnik BR. Risk of radiocontrast nephropathy in patients with and without diabetes mellitus. *Kidney Int* 1994; **45**:259–65.

2. Stone GW, McCullough PA, Tumlin JA et al. Fenoldopam mesylate for the prevention of contrast-induced nephropathy: a randomized controlled trial. *JAMA* 2003; **290**:2284–91.

3. Kurnik BR, Weisberg LS, Cuttler IM, Kurnik PB. Effects of atrial natriuretic peptide versus mannitol on renal blood flow during radiocontrast infusion in chronic renal failure. *J Lab Clin Med* 1990; **116**:27–36.

4. Wang A, Holcslaw T, Bashore T et al. Exacerbation of radiocontrast nephrotoxicity by endothelin receptor antagonism. *Kidney Int* 2000; **57**:1675–80.

5. Khoury Z, Schlicht J, Como J et al. The effect of prophylactic nifedipine on renal function in patients administered contrast media. *Pharmacotherapy* 1995; **15**:59–65.

6. Liss P. Effects of contrast media on renal microcirculation and oxygen tension. An experimental study in the rat. *Acta Radiol Suppl* 1997; **409**:1–29.

7. Nygren A, Ulfendahl HR, Hansell P, Erikson U. Effects of intravenous contrast media on cortical and medullary blood flow in the rat kidney. *Invest Radiol* 1988; **23**:753–61.

8. Heyman S, Rosenberger C, Rosen S. Regional alterations in renal haemodynamics and oxygenation: a role in contrast medium-induced nephropathy. *Nephrol Dial Transplant* 2005; **20(Suppl 1)**:i6–i11.

9. Brezis M, Rosen S. Hypoxia of the renal medulla: its implications for disease. *N Engl J Med* 1995; **332**:647–55.

10. Agmon Y, Peleg H, Greenfeld Z, Rosen S, Brezis M. Nitric oxide and prostanoids protect the renal outer medulla from radiocontrast toxicity in the rat. *J Clin Invest* 1994; **94**:1069–75.

11. Heyman SN, Brezis M, Epstein FH et al. Early renal medullary hypoxic injury from radiocontrast and indomethacin. *Kidney Int* 1991; **40**:632–42.

12. Heyman SN, Brezis M, Reubinoff CA et al. Acute renal failure with selective medullary injury in the rat. *J Clin Invest* 1988; **82**:401–12.

13. Tervahartiala P, Kivisaari R, Vehmans T, Virtanen I. Structural changes in the renal proximal tubular cells induced by iodinated contrast media. *Nephron* 1997; **76**:96–102.

14. Han W, Bailly V, Abichandani R, Thadani R. Kidney injury molecule-1 (KIM-1): a novel biomarker for human renal proximal tubule injury. *Kidney Int* 2002; **62**:237–44.

15. Colucci WS, Elkayam U, Horton DP et al. Intravenous nesiritide, a natriuretic peptide, in the treatment of decompensated congestive heart failure. Nesiritide Study Group. *N Engl J Med* 2000; **343**:246–53.

16. Mathur VS, Swan SK, Lambrecht LJ et al. The effects of fenoldopam, a selective dopamine receptor agonist, on systemic and renal hemodynamics in normotensive subjects. *Crit Care Med* 1999; **27**:1832–7.

17. Tumlin J, Wang A, Murray P, Mathur V. Fenoldopam mesylate blocks reductions in renal plasma flow following radiocontrast dye infusion: a pilot trial in the prevention of contrast nephropathy. *Am Heart J* 2002; **143**:894–903.

18. Garwood S, Hines R. Perioperative renal preservation: dopexamine and fenoldopam – new agents to augment renal performance. *Semin Anesth Periop Med Pain* 1998; **17**:308–18.

19. Adams KF Jr, Mathur VS, Gheorghiade M. B-type natriuretic peptide: from bench to bedside. *Am Heart J* 2003; **145(2 Suppl)**:S34–46.

20. Allgren RL, Marbury TC, Rahman SN et al. Anaritide in acute tubular necrosis. Auriculin Anaritide Acute Renal Failure Study Group. *N Engl J Med* 1997; **336**:828–34.

21. Chen HH, Lainchbury JG, Burnett JC. Natriuretic peptide receptors and neutral endopeptidase in mediating the renal actions of a new therapeutic synthetic natriuretic peptide dendroaspis natriuretic peptide. *J Am Coll Cardiol* 2002; **40**:1186–91.

22. Gottlieb S, Brater D, Thomas I et al. BG9719 (CVT-124), an A1 adenosine receptor antagonist, protects against the decline in renal function observed with diuretic therapy. *Circulation* 2002; **106**:1348–53.

23. Mitchell A, Luckebergfeld B, Buhrmann S et al. Effects of systemic endothelin A receptor antagonism in various vascular beds in men: in vivo interactions of the major blood pressure-regulating systems and associations with the GNB3 C825T polymorphism. *Clin Pharmacol Ther* 2004; **5**:396–408.

24. Koch JA, Plum J, Grabensee B, Modder U. Prostaglandin E1: a new agent for the prevention of renal dysfunction in high risk patients caused by radiocontrast media? PGE1 Study Group. *Nephrol Dial Transplant* 2000; **15**:43–9.

25. Persson PB, Patzak A. Renal haemodynamic alterations in contrast medium-induced nephropathy and the benefit of hydration. *Nephrol Dial Transplant* 2005; **20(Suppl 1)**:i2–i5.

26. Merten GJ, Burgess WP, Gray LV et al. Prevention of contrast-induced nephropathy with sodium bicarbonate: a randomized controlled trial. *JAMA* 2004; **291**:2328–34.

27. Tepel M, van der Giet M, Schwarzfeld C et al. Prevention of radiographic-contrast-agent-induced reductions in renal function by acetylcysteine [see comments]. *N Engl J Med* 2000; **343**:180–4.

28. Shusterman NH, Elliott WJ, White WB. Fenoldopam, but not nitroprusside, improves renal function in severely hypertensive patients with impaired renal function. *Am J Med* 1993; **95**:161–8.

29. Kien ND, Moore PG, Jaffe RS. Cardiovascular function during induced hypotension by fenoldopam or sodium nitroprusside in anesthetized dogs. *Anesth Analg* 1992; **74**:72–8.

30. O'Connell D, Ragsdale V, Boyd D, Felder R, Carey R. Differential human renal tubular responses to dopamine type 1 receptor stimulation are determined by blood pressure status. *Hypertension* 1997; **29**:115–22.

31. Bakris GL, Lass NA, Glock D. Renal hemodynamics in radiocontrast medium-induced renal dysfunction: a role for dopamine-1 receptors. *Kidney Int* 1999; **56**:206–10.

32. Tumlin JA, Dunbar LM, Oparil S et al. Fenoldopam, a dopamine agonist, for hypertensive emergency: a multicenter randomized trial. Fenoldopam Study Group. *Acad Emerg Med* 2000; **7**:653–62.

33. Chamsuddin AA, Kowalik KJ, Bjarnason H et al. Using a dopamine type 1A receptor agonist in high-risk patients to ameliorate contrast-associated nephropathy. *AJR* 2002; **179**:591–6.

34. Madyoon H, Croushore L, Weaver D, Mathur V. Use of fenoldopam to prevent radiocontrast nephropathy in high-risk patients. *Cathet Cardiovasc Interven* 2001; **53**:341–5.

35. Stone GW, McCullough PA, Tumlin JA et al. Fenoldopam mesylate for the prevention of contrast-induced nephropathy: a randomized controlled trial. *JAMA* 2003; **290**:2284–91.

36. Mathur V, Teirstein P, Patel S, Valencia A, Goodson B. Evidence for reduced systemic exposure to fenoldopam following local renal delivery compared to intravenous delivery. *Blood Purif* 2004; **22**:38.

37. Mathur V, Teirstein P, Anderson E, Croushore L, Maydoon H. Targeted renal drug delivery with fenoldopam: a multicenter, randomized, controlled trial. *J Am Soc Nephrol* 2004; **15**:346A.

38. Grube E, Teirstein P, Baim D et al. Intra-renal fenoldopam increases renal artery flow velocity and causes less effects on blood pressure lowering than intravenous fenoldopam. *Am J Cardiol* 2004; **94**:176E.

39. Cohen MG, Fearon W, Weisz G et al. Use of a new bifurcated renal infusion catheter for clinical management of high risk angiography patients: data from the Be-RITe! National Registry. In: *Cardiovascular Revascularization Therapeutics*; March 28–31 2005; Washington DC, 2005.

40. Mathur V, Goodson B, Patel S, Valencia A, Elkins J. Evidence for substantial renal first pass effects of human B-type natriuretic peptide (nesiritide) following intra-renal infusion. *J Cardiac Fail* 2004; **10**:S68.

12. MAGNETIC RESONANCE AND CARBON DIOXIDE ANGIOGRAPHY IN IMAGING AND INTERVENTIONS

Günther Schneider and Roland Seidel

Contrast-agent-induced nephropathy is currently an important area of interest and discussion among the radiologic community. Possible alternatives to conventional X-ray angiography and other more recent techniques that utilize iodinated contrast agents and ionizing radiation (computed tomographic angiography [CTA], rotational angiography) are unenhanced and contrast-enhanced magnetic resonance angiography (MRA), at least in the field of diagnostic imaging. This chapter will discuss the different techniques for MRA and the characteristics of the currently available magnetic resonance (MR) contrast agents for contrast-enhanced MRA in today's established indications. Additionally, new approaches for MR guided vascular interventions will be presented. Finally, a brief review of the clinical performance and interpretation of carbon dioxide (CO_2) digital subtraction angiography will be provided.

Unenhanced and contrast-enhanced MRA

Techniques for unenhanced MR angiography

In conventional X-ray angiography, administration of contrast agent is necessary in order to depict the blood vessels. After arterial catheterization and injection of an iodinated contrast agent, two-dimensional projection images of the lumen of the vessel are acquired from chosen angles. For every new projection this procedure has to be repeated. The availability of three-dimensional rotational angiography and CTA may help to overcome the issue of repeated acquisitions inherent in conventional X-ray angiography, but at the expense of high radiation doses and increased doses of iodinated contrast agents.

Unenhanced MRA differs from conventional X-ray angiography (digital subtraction angiography [DSA] and other angiographic techniques) in that blood vessels are depicted non-invasively in the absence of contrast agent injection. Unenhanced MR techniques allow the acquisition of three-dimensional datasets or stacks of two-dimensional images that contain all vessels in the volume of interest. The acquired images included in the three-dimensional dataset are called 'source images' (Figure 12.1). Projectional angiographic displays of the vessel are subsequently reconstructed from the data using the maximum intensity projection (MIP) postprocessing algorithm (Figure 12.2), which generates angiogram-like images from the entire dataset or a subset from any desired viewing angle without the need for further measurement. Another advantage of unenhanced MRA versus X-ray angiography derives from the fact that extravascular tissue is depicted together with the vessels, thereby allowing the correlation of blood flow abnormalities with associated soft tissue pathologies.

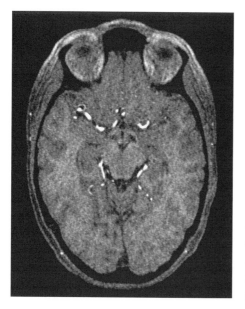

Figure 12.1 *Source image of an unenhanced two-dimensional time-of-flight MR angiography examination of cerebral vasculature. Due to flow effects, the arterial vessels are displayed with high signal intensity. A stack of axial images was used to make the maximum intensity projections demonstrated in Figure 12.2.*

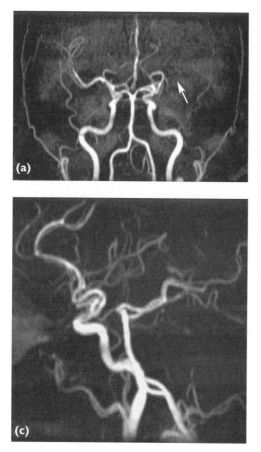

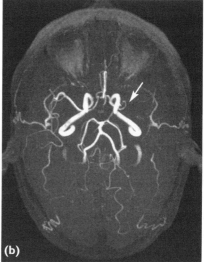

Figure 12.2 *Unenhanced time-of-flight MR angiography. (a) to (c) Maximum intensity projection reconstructions of the cerebral vasculature in different projections, calculated from an axial two-dimensional raw data set. Note the absence of the right medial cerebral artery distal to the M1 segment (arrow in (a) and (b)) in a patient with acute stroke.*

Unenhanced MRA comprises those MR techniques that rely solely on flow effects. Unlike contrast-enhanced MRA and X-ray angiography, which depict the vessel lumen filled with contrast agent, it is just the movement of blood that is seen in the unenhanced MR angiogram.

One striking phenomenon in MRA is the effect of blood flow. Typically, flowing blood produces a hyperintense signal while the background signal from stationary tissue remains largely suppressed ('bright-blood' angiography). In unenhanced MRA there are basically two approaches to performing 'bright-blood' vessel imaging: time-of-flight (TOF) and phase-contrast (PC) angiography.

Clinical applications of unenhanced MRA

In today's clinical practice, unenhanced MRA techniques are mainly employed for the imaging of intracranial vasculature. In this territory, they are established as screening methods that allow good-quality visualization of the vascular anatomy. Typical high-resolution measurements require less than 5 minutes and thus can be performed routinely in patients with suspected intracranial vascular disease. Although unenhanced techniques may also be applied to imaging of blood vessels in vascular territories outside the central nervous system (CNS) (Figure 12.3), contrast-enhanced

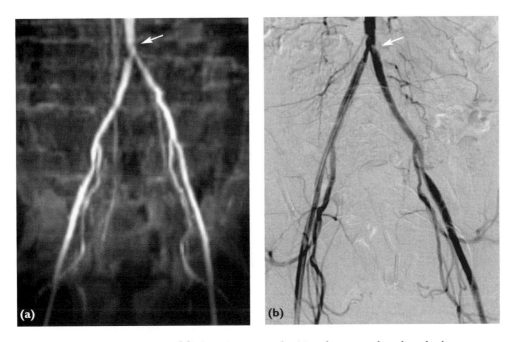

Figure 12.3 *Unenhanced time-of-flight MR angiography (a) and corresponding digital subtraction angiography (DSA) (b) in a patient with atherosclerotic stenosis of the aorta bifurcation. Although the unenhanced maximum intensity projection reconstruction of a time-of-flight MR angiography depicts the stenosis (arrow) sufficiently to make a diagnosis and shows good correlation with the DSA (arrow), the long acquisition time (> 8 min) and relatively poor resolution render this unenhanced technique inappropriate for diagnostic work-up in patients with suspected stenosis of the run-off vessels.*

MRA is now firmly established as the dominating approach in the extracranial and peripheral regions in large part due to the considerably shorter imaging times that contrast-enhanced MRA requires in these territories.

An exception to the slight interest of using unenhanced imaging outside the CNS is visualization of the coronary arteries. Several studies have suggested that unenhanced MRA may have great potential for imaging the coronary vessels. However, there is still no consensus as to whether contrast-enhanced or unenhanced techniques will be the preferred imaging method in the future. Unfortunately, a series of major problems has to be overcome before coronary MRA and acquisition of coronary vessel wall data can be performed successfully in routine practice. The heart is subject to both extrinsic and intrinsic motion due to breathing and its natural periodic contraction. Both these motion components exceed the dimensions of the coronary arteries, resulting in the need for efficient motion suppression techniques if satisfactory acquisition of coronary MR data is to be achieved in the submillimeter range. ECG gating is absolutely essential in coronary MRA to offset the intrinsic cardiac motion, while either breath-hold or navigator techniques that register the motion of the diaphragm are needed to compensate for respiratory motion. A major drawback of breath-hold techniques derives from the fact that patients are typically unable to hold their breaths for sufficient time. Consequently, the resolution of images has to be reduced if the coverage is not sufficient. Unfortunately, a consequence of reduced resolution is often insufficient image quality for diagnosis. To overcome the limitations associated with breath holding, different methods such as MR navigators[1] have been developed to allow for free-breathing coronary MRA. However, even though great progress has been made with regard to motion suppression, MR imaging hardware, software, and scanning protocols, the spatial resolution achievable with MRA is still inferior to that obtainable with X-ray coronary angiography. While an improvement in spatial resolution is always accompanied by a trade-off in terms of signal-to-noise ratio (SNR), this may partly be overcome by the use of high-field systems[2] and contrast agents.[3]

With MR contrast agents, the T1 relaxation of blood can be shortened, allowing for increased contrast-to-noise ratio (CNR) for coronary MRA.[4,5] The contrast agents currently available for coronary MRA are the traditional extracellular gadolinium (Gd)-based agents. However, because extracellular agents quickly extravasate into the extravascular space, their use requires rapid first-pass imaging, thereby necessitating breath holding.[6] This basically results in the same problems as already mentioned for unenhanced approaches to coronary artery imaging. Furthermore, first-pass coronary MRA with extravascular contrast agents is also limited by the need for repeated contrast injections since imaging of the coronary arteries requires more than one three-dimensional dataset. With each subsequent injection, the CNR will decrease as the signal from the extracellular space continuously increases following initial contrast administration.

An attempt to overcome the inherent limitations of extracellular contrast agents is the development of intravascular agents (the so-called 'blood-pool agents') based either on Gd or iron oxide particles.[7] The use of intravascular agents has the advantage of allowing image acquisition over a longer period of time after intravenous administration of the contrast agent (Figure 12.4). Thus, non-breath-hold techniques can be employed, and repeated scans have similar CNR values, thereby obviating the need for repeated injections. Furthermore, since only very small doses of contrast are administered, the use of intravascular agents is more appropriate in patients with renal insufficiency. More detailed discussion of contrast agents and techniques for contrast-enhanced MRA will follow in subsequent sections.

166

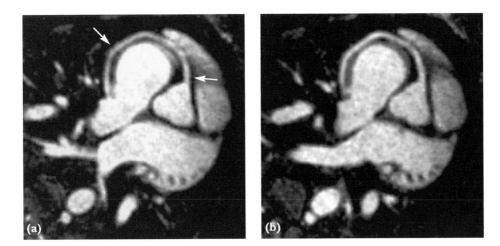

Figure 12.4   *Coronary MR angiography 2 min (a) and 40 min (b) after injection of an intravascular MR contrast agent (B 22956, Bracco Imaging SpA, Milan, Italy). The maximum intensity projection images at 2 min and 40 min postinjection depict the right coronary artery (arrows) with a high signal-to-noise ratio and without significant loss of signal.*

In summary, because of its non-invasive nature, three-dimensional imaging capabilities, and suitability for soft tissue characterization, MRA appears to be a potentially powerful modality for both coronary lumen and vessel wall imaging. However, at present coronary MRA cannot be considered as a routine imaging modality in patients with coronary artery disease because of the lack of image quality reproducibility and problems associated with the acquisition of adequate image sets. Moreover, the need for dedicated scanners and experienced staff further hampers the widespread use of this technique.

On the other hand, with further technologic refinements, improvements of the spatial resolution on high-field MR scanners, and evolution towards a push-bottom technique, there is hope of significantly improving the ability to detect and even characterize the tissue and plaque components of the vessel wall in diseased coronary arteries. This may have far reaching implications for the management of patients with established coronary heart disease and may, in some cases, replace some of the currently established imaging modalities.

Contrast-enhanced MRA

In recent years, contrast-enhanced MRA has emerged as a technique of choice for diagnostic vascular imaging.[8,9] Technical improvements in contrast-enhanced MRA over the past decade have significantly improved not only image quality but also image acquisition speed, reliability, and ease of use. Using traditional extracellular Gd-based contrast agents, contrast-enhanced MRA yields angiographic data comparable to – and in some instances superior to – those of conventional catheter angiography. Contrast-enhanced MRA, moreover, is non-invasive and has inherent clinical benefits compared to catheter X-ray angiography and CTA in that there is no exposure to ionizing radiation or nephrotoxic effect of iodinated contrast media. Nephrotoxicity is a major issue in patients with vascular disease as many also have diabetes mellitus and/or renal insufficiency, making the use of iodinated contrast agents undesirable. The availability of contrast-enhanced MRA may therefore limit the utilization of iodinated contrast media to vascular interventions.

Contrast-enhanced MRA relies on the T1 shortening effect of Gd-chelate contrast agents in blood. This is different from the time of flight (TOF) and phase contrast (PC) techniques used in MRA, which exploit the inherent motion of blood flow to generate a vascular signal. By relying on the presence of a contrast agent within the vessel lumen, the vascular signal obtained by contrast-enhanced MRA is not hampered by the flow-related artifacts (i.e. slow flow or signal loss from spin saturation) that can degrade flow-based MRA techniques and often result in overestimation of stenosis severity or even simulation of vascular occlusion.[10]

With contrast-enhanced MRA, arteries will be visualized if image acquisition is performed during the arterial phase of the contrast bolus. If, on the other hand, imaging is delayed during the venous phase of the bolus, veins will be visualized. As in conventional angiography, imaging a contrast agent during its vascular transit enables the generation of a 'luminogram'. Since vascular enhancement is a transient and dynamic process, the critical element for contrast-enhanced MRA, as with catheter-based X-ray angiography, is timing of the imaging. Data from contrast-enhanced MRA can be postprocessed to yield projections very similar to those of conventional catheter angiography (Figure 12.5). Contrast-enhanced MRA, generally performed using three-dimensional MRA pulse sequences, has the added benefit of yielding volumetric datasets, which can also be postprocessed using multiplanar reformation and various three-dimensional visualization techniques, notably maximum intensity projection (MIP) and volume-rendered (VR) display (Figure 12.6). These methods often enable superior appreciation of vascular segments in question that would otherwise be obscured by overlying structures and overlapping vessels on planar projections of conventional catheter angiography.

Over the past decade, contrast-enhanced MRA has benefited from numerous improvements in scanner hardware and from the development of specialized contrast-enhanced MRA software. As a result, it has progressively evolved into the technique of choice for evaluating many – if not most – vascular beds, such as the carotid arteries (Figure 12.7),[11] the aorta,[12] the renal arteries (Figure 12.8),[13] and the peripheral vasculature (Figure 12.9).[14]

The fact that contrast-enhanced MRA can today replace catheter angiography in diagnostic imaging of most vascular territories may limit the use of iodinated contrast media to interventional procedures. Thus, this imaging modality offers a strategy to decrease the risk of contrast-induced nephropathy, especially in patients with pre-existing renal insufficiency.

Contrast agents for contrast-enhanced mR Angiography

On one hand, largely due to advances in hard- and software design, techniques and applications for contrast-enhanced MRA have developed rapidly in recent years. On the other hand, the advent of innovative new contrast agents with properties distinct from those of the traditional, extracellular Gd agents promises to further expand the clinical applicability of contrast-enhanced MRA, making this the modality of choice for diagnostic imaging of the vasculature.

With few exceptions, most of the commercially available contrast agents are not approved directly for contrast-enhanced MRA.[15] Gd chelates, which have demonstrated their clinical usefulness in improving the detection of various neoplastic, inflammatory, and functional abnormalities of a variety of organs, are the most widely used agents. These extracellular, non-specific

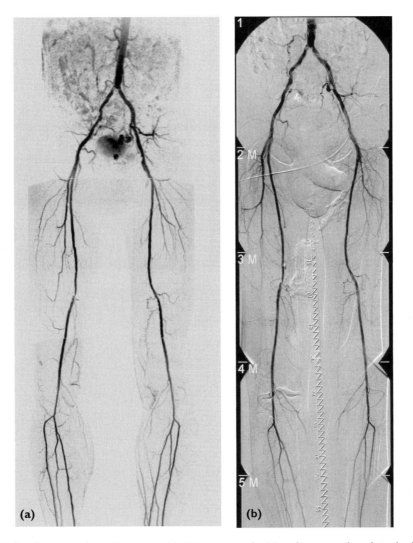

Figure 12.5 *Contrast-enhanced moving-table MR angiography (a) and corresponding digital subtraction angiography (DSA) (b) in a patient with peripheral arterial disease. For MR angiography, a total dose of 0.1 mmol/kg body weight of gadobenate dimeglumine (Gd-BOPTA, Bracco Imaging SpA, Milan, Italy), which corresponds to a total volume of 14 ml, was administered intravenously. Note the excellent correlation between the MR angiography and the DSA. Because of the diagnostic value of these images, the injection of an iodinated contrast medium may be avoided for the evaluation of peripheral arterial disease.*

contrast agents distribute in a manner comparable to the distribution of iodinated contrast media. Their use for many clinical indications is justified because, in conjunction with improved imaging techniques, they are safe and provide additional morphologic and functional information compared with unenhanced imaging.

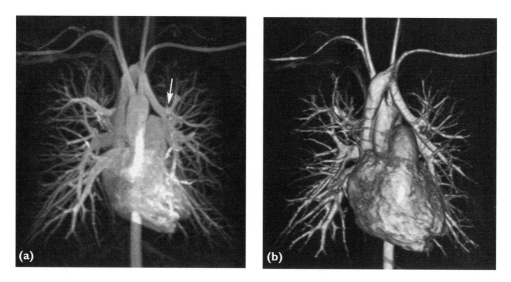

Figure 12.6 *Comparison between maximum intensity projection reconstruction (MIP) (a) and volume-rendering technique (b) in the evaluation of anomalous venous return by contrast-enhanced MRA in a pediatric patient. Although the MIP reconstruction already depicts the anomalous return of the veins of the left upper lobe ((a), arrow) into a so-called vertical vein, the volume-rendered image (b) better depicts the anatomic relationship between the different vascular structures and may help to plan surgery.*

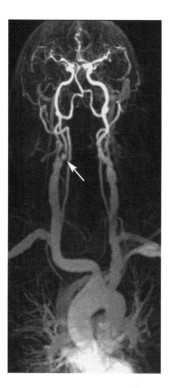

Figure 12.7 *Contrast-enhanced MR angiography of the carotid arteries. Excellent non-invasive depiction of the supra-aortic vessels in a patient with advanced aterosclerotic disease and depiction of a high-grade stenosis of the right internal carotid artery (arrow).*

170

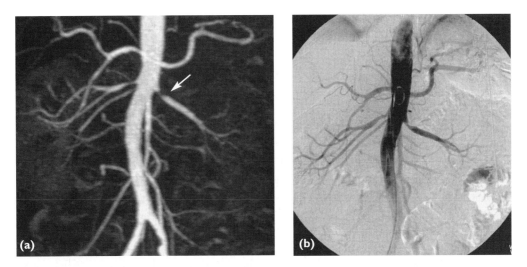

Figure 12.8 *Contrast-enhanced MR angiography (a) and corresponding digital subtraction angiography (b) of the abdominal aorta in a patient with suspected renal artery stenosis. Note the excellent correlation between the two techniques in depicting a high-grade stenosis (arrow) of the left renal artery and a moderate stenosis of the right renal artery.*

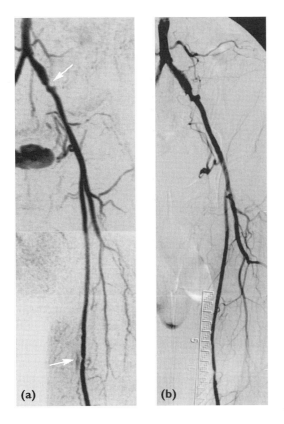

Figure 12.9 *Details of an examination of the run-off vessels by means of contrast-enhanced MR angiography (a) and digital subtraction angiography (b). Excellent correlation between the two techniques in depicting multiple stenoses (arrows in (a)) of the left iliac and superficial femoral arteries is apparent.*

171

Gd chelates are extremely well tolerated at both standard (0.1 mmol/kg body weight, ~0.2 ml/kg) and higher doses (up to 0.3 mmol/kg body weight), with no clinically relevant differences among the disparate agents available today.[16,17] Single adverse events occur with a frequency of approximately 1% or less in all patients. Non-ionic complexes with low osmolality were developed to improve tolerance and allow the use of higher doses. However, because of the low amounts of compounds injected for MR imaging, the ionic charge of ionic Gd complexes is not a crucial factor. Furthermore, the increased plasma osmolality following administration of Gd chelates is very low, unlike that which is observed following administration of iodinated contrast media. Indeed, from a safety viewpoint, it is inappropriate to compare ionic and non-ionic MR imaging contrast agents in the same way that ionic and non-ionic X-ray contrast media are compared.[18]

Gd chelates are excreted unchanged by passive glomerular filtration and the package insert information provided by manufacturers usually indicates that 'caution should be exercised in patients with severely impaired renal function' or 'as there are no studies with the contrast agent in patients with impaired renal function, its use cannot be recommended for this group of patients'. However, several studies suggest that Gd chelates are well tolerated in patients with renal insufficiency. No significant change of serum creatinine levels was observed in patients with moderate or severe impairment of renal function after the administration of 0.1 mmol/kg gadopentetate dimeglumine (Gd-DTPA) or gadoterate meglumine (Gd-DOTA).[19,20] Similarly, gadobutrol (1 mol/l) at a dose of 0.1 or 0.3 mmol/kg proved to be a safe MR contrast agent in a study of 21 patients with impaired renal function.[21] Gd chelates can be eliminated by dialysis, with more than 95% of the administered dose being removed by the third dialysis session.[21] Indeed, in patients with chronic renal failure on hemodialysis, Gd chelates are efficiently cleared. The mean half-life of the plasma concentration of Gd-DTPA is 1.87 ± 0.71 hours in patients on dialysis, which is comparable to the value obtained for patients with normal renal function. According to a study conducted by Yoshikawa and Davies,[22] gadoteridol at a dose of 0.3 mmol/kg body weight could be safely administered to patients with endstage renal disease on dialysis. Tombach et al[23] documented the safety and dialysability of gadobutrol at doses of 0.1 and 0.3 mmol/kg body weight. They showed that the mean eliminated fraction increased from 68.2 ± 12.7 to $98.0\pm1.8\%$, respectively, after one three-hour haemodialysis session.

New contrast agents for MRA

As mentioned previously, non-protein-binding Gd chelates have been the agents primarily used for MR angiography. Modified paramagnetic Gd-based agents with varying degrees of protein interaction have been developed, and these, together with new superparamagnetic compounds, are currently under clinical evaluation for use as blood-pool contrast agents.

It is likely that two different types of contrast agent will soon be available: extracellular agents for first-pass MRA and intravascular agents mainly for steady-state MRA. The so-called paramagnetic 'blood-pool' contrast agents are agents for which the intravascular residence time is considerably extended compared to the conventional 'first-pass' Gd agents. With these agents, the intravascular signal remains high for an extended period of time, thereby permitting not only conventional first-pass contrast-enhanced MRA, but also MR imaging during a more prolonged 'steady-state' time frame. As mentioned above, a primary indication would be coronary artery imaging. However, these agents may also be of interest for vascular imaging during interventions since no repeated injection of contrast agent would be needed to depict the vessels with fast, real-time imaging sequences.

There are two principal types of paramagnetic 'blood-pool' contrast agent: those whose intravascular residence time is prolonged due to the capability of the Gd chelate for strong interaction with serum proteins, and those that have a macromolecular structure whose large size limits the extent of extravasation compared to the first-pass Gd agents. Of these macromolecular agents, both paramagnetic Gd-based agents and superparamagnetic iron-oxide-based agents are available. However, none of these agents is yet approved for clinical use.

MR-guided vascular interventions – current status and future perspectives

Even though X-ray fluoroscopy still is the imaging modality of choice to guide vascular interventions, MR imaging has been receiving increasing attention in recent years, in particular because of the perception that MRA is now a serious alternative to DSA for diagnostic vascular imaging. A serious drawback of X-ray fluoroscopy is the potential radiation hazard for patients and operators, since some interventions can take up to several hours. In addition, this method relies on the injection of iodinated contrast medium with the known contraindications and adverse effects on renal function.

A few years ago, the application of MR imaging to guide vascular interventional procedures was not considered feasible. Two technological advances have occurred since that time. First, the development of open or short-bore MR imaging systems has facilitated the performance of MR-guided interventions. Second, contrast-enhanced MRA has become established in clinical routine with the introduction of fast measurement techniques.[24] However, MR-guided vascular interventions require real-time visualization of catheters and guide wires to define their location with regards to the vascular system and surrounding tissues.

One of the most challenging applications of endovascular MRI is the treatment of vessel stenosis by percutaneous transluminal angioplasty (PTA). The feasibility of MR-guided PTA was demonstrated in animal models using passive tracking of catheters in the abdominal aorta[25] and renal arteries. More recently, patient studies have been performed. Manke et al evaluated MR-guided stent placement in 14 iliac artery stenoses and found the procedure to be feasible, although time consuming, and not yet ready for clinical use.[26]

One of the important needs in performing MR-guided endovascular interventions is the repetitive visualization of the vessel segments of interest. This requires either repeated intra-arterial injections of the contrast agent, with the likelihood of the limits mandated by the regulatory authorities being exceeded, or the use of intravascular agents that are not yet approved. Recently, several investigators have demonstrated that the intra-arterial low-dose application of Gd-based contrast material is feasible and provides optimal signal enhancement of the vessel lumen during interventions in animals.[27]

Another approach in interventions would be, as already mentioned, the use of intravascular or blood-pool agents that allow for visualization of vessels for a longer time following administration. An animal study in pigs has shown that one intravenous injection of SH U 555 C, an iron-oxide-based blood-pool agent, enables long, continuous intravascular signal intensity (SI) enhancement during MRA, and, in combination with susceptibility artifact-based device tracking, allows the performance of MR-guided intravascular interventions in an open MR imaging system.[28]

Recently, Serfaty et al demonstrated the feasibility of MRI-guided coronary artery catheterization and balloon angioplasty inflation in normal coronary arteries in dogs.[29] They state, as other investigators did in previous published studies, that with future improvements in MR-imaging technology and intravascular antenna design, interventional MRI may facilitate treatments of coronary artery and heart disease, and provide new imaging possibilities without the need for ionizing radiation or iodinated contrast agents. Unfortunately, MR-guided vascular interventions are still not feasible at present, even though the basics for a new imaging technique for percutaneous vascular therapy have been established.

In summary, MRA can today be considered a viable alternative to catheter-based angiography in diagnostic imaging of most vascular territories. Drawbacks are still apparent in imaging of the coronaries, but with the tremendous progress seen in recent years one can foresee that even routine MR imaging of the coronary arteries will be possible in the near future. Although MR-guided vascular interventions are not yet ready for clinical use, this too may change in the not too distant future.

CO_2 digital subtraction angiography

Carbon dioxide has been used as a vascular contrast agent since the 1950s, when it was first administered for the diagnosis of pericardial effusions and later for depiction of venous structures within the liver.[30] Since that time, the use of CO_2 as an alternative to iodinated contrast media in angiographic procedures has grown. It is now used for a variety of angiographic investigations below the diaphragm in both the arterial and venous circulations. A principal advantage is its safety profile: CO_2 is neither allergenic nor nephrotoxic.

The reported incidence of contrast-induced nephropathy in patients with underlying chronic renal insufficiency varies from 9% to 93% after administration of iodinated contrast material.[31,32] This variability reflects the use of different criteria for the definition of contrast-induced nephropathy as well as differences in the patient populations studied. Moreover, a variety of different pre- and postinterventional algorithms for contrast media applications have been reported.[31,33] The non-allergenic and non-nephrotoxic characteristics of CO_2 make it an ideal contrast agent for patients with a history of severe allergic reaction to iodinated contrast media, underlying renal insufficiency or diabetes. The accuracy of this angiographic contrast agent in a variety of diagnostic applications is well established and no evidence of false-negative studies has been reported.[30,34]

For many years, CO_2 was injected manually, which often resulted in insufficient image quality and poor filling of arterial vessels.[35] As a consequence, only a few comparative studies with conventional angiography have been performed.[36,37] The development of specifically designed CO_2 injectors that avoid the risk of an explosive effect during injection rapidly permitted constant doses to be delivered without contamination by room air. On this basis, the first retrospective study of 128 CO_2 arteriograms of the lower extremity was published by Seeger et al.[38] In this study, good to excellent image quality and a high diagnostic correlation (95%) between the CO_2 angiographic studies and conventional angiographies were described (Figure 12.10). Similar results were obtained with CO_2 angiography of the lower extremities by other authors, confirming the potential diagnostic value of this imaging modality.[39,40] Unfortunately, in contrast to these

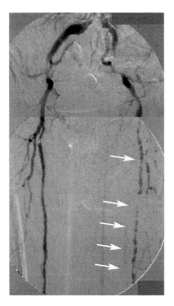

Figure 12.10 *Carbon dioxide arteriography of the lower extremity. Although the iliac arteries are imaged with sufficient resolution, the left superficial femoral artery shows multiple artificial stenoses (arrows), most likely attributable to a fragmentation of the gas column.*

promising results, several other authors found only limited diagnostic efficacy of CO_2, especially for the evaluation of the infrapopliteal vascular region: incomplete or inconclusive examinations occurred in about 50% of investigations.[41,42] These findings were attributed in large part to a fragmentation of the column of gas in the peripheral vascular segments (Figure 12.10). For those cases in which complete investigations were possible, mild to significant overestimations of stenosis were observed compared to iodinated angiography. This was attributed to incomplete gas filling of the vessel.[41]

Another critical aspect of this procedure is the marked discomfort experienced by most of the patients. Many authors have invariably reported higher levels of discomfort when employing CO_2 compared to iodinated contrast agents due to the rapid release of large volumes of gas into the abdominal aorta that causes strong abdominal pain. As a consequence, cramps, nausea, vomiting, etc. can occur and may limit this diagnostic approach.[39,40,42]

The main complication in using CO_2 as a contrast agent for injection into the abdominal aorta is intestinal ischemia. This is most likely caused by the collection of entrapped gas within the mesenteric vessels. Abdominal pain, vomiting, diarrhea, and even intestinal infarction and necrosis may occur.[43] Pain of the lower limbs is caused by a similar mechanism within the peripheral vascular regions.

Another field for the application of this technique is renal angiography. In a series of 47 patients published by Beese et al, 79% of the angiographic studies performed with CO_2 were diagnostic.[44] The diagnostic results were in agreement with the results of another study that compared CO_2 with iodinated contrast media in renal angiography.[45] In a minority of the cases, an adjunctive administration of an iodinated or Gd-based contrast medium was necessary for accurate evaluation of vessel structures. The use of CO_2 as a contrast agent for vascular interventional procedures (Figure 12.11) has also been described.[46–48] However, reliable demonstration of successful coil

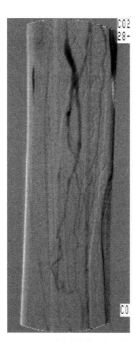

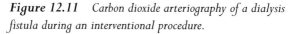

Figure 12.11   *Carbon dioxide arteriography of a dialysis fistula during an interventional procedure.*

positioning in cases of vascular embolization is problematic since occlusion detection with CO_2 is very poor. Moreover, the use of CO_2 would be inappropriate when particulate or liquid embolic agents are injected.[46]

The application of CO_2 has also been reported for the evaluation of venous structures. For the diagnostic approach of portal or splenic veins, a puncture of the spleen with a 25 or 27 gauge needle can be performed enabling spleno-portography.[49,50] However, since the reported patient numbers in the literature are limited, further prospective studies need to be performed to reliably assess the diagnostic accuracy of this method.

The use of CO_2 in the liver is well established. Due to its low viscosity, rapid diffusion through the hepatic sinusoids is possible, permitting wedged hepatic portography. In this setting it can be used for the guidance of transjugular intrahepatic portosystemic shunt transjugular intrahepatic portosystemic shunt (TIPS) procedures.[51]

In summary, the use of CO_2 as an alternative arterial or venous contrast agent is possible for many diagnostic studies of vascular structures below the diaphragm. In cases of incompletely contrasted vessels, an adjunctive administration of an iodinated or Gd-based contrast agent can be performed. Compared to conventional angiography, patient discomfort is higher with CO_2 and leads more often to premature termination of the diagnostic procedure. Moreover, gas entrapment can lead to adverse effects and may even result in tissue necrosis in rare cases. Finally, ascending gas into cerebral structures can have neurotoxic effects. Therefore, the use of this alternative contrast agent should be restricted to patients with contraindications to conventional iodinated contrast media and should be used only for imaging below the diaphragm.

References

1. Ehman RL, Felmlee JP. Adaptive technique for high-definition MR imaging of moving structures. *Radiology* 1989; **173**:255–63.

2. Stuber M, Botnar RM, Fischer SE et al. Preliminary report on in vivo coronary MRA at 3 Tesla in humans. *Magn Reson Med* 2002; **48**:425–9.

3. Huber ME, Paetsch I, Schnackenburg B et al. Performance of a new gadolinium-based intravascular contrast agent in free-breathing inversion-recovery 3D coronary MRA. *Magn Reson Med* 2003; **49**:115–21.

4. Hofman MBM, Henson RE, Kovacs SJ et al. Blood pool agent strongly improves 3D magnetic resonance coronary angiography using an inversion pre-pulse. *Magn Reson Med* 1999; **41**:360–7.

5. Stuber M, Botnar RM, Danias PG et al. Contrast agent-enhanced, free-breathing, three-dimensional coronary magnetic resonance angiography. *J Magn Reson Imaging* 1999; **10**:790–9.

6. Goldfarb JW, Edelman RR. Coronary arteries: breath-hold, gadolinium-enhanced, three-dimensional MR angiography. *Radiology* 1998; **206**:830–4.

7. Li D, Dolan RP, Walovitch RC, Lauffer RB. Three-dimensional MRI of coronary arteries using an intravascular contrast agent. *Magn Reson Med* 1998; **39**:1014–18.

8. Koelemay MJ, Lijmer JG, Stoker J et al. Magnetic resonance angiography for the evaluation of lower extremity arterial disease. A meta-analysis. *JAMA* 2001; **285**:1338–45.

9. Yucel EK, Anderson CM, Edelman RR et al. AHA scientific statement. Magnetic resonance angiography: update on applications for extracranial arteries. *Circulation* 1999; **100**:2284–301.

10. Kaufman JA, McCarter D, Geller SC et al. Two-dimensional time-of-flight MR angiography of the lower extremities: artifacts and pitfalls. *AJR* 1998; **171**:129–35.

11. Huston J 3rd, Fain SB, Wald JT et al. Carotid artery: elliptic centric contrast-enhanced MR angiography compared with conventional angiography. *Radiology* 2001; **218**:138–43.

12. Ho VB, Corse WR, Hood MN, Rowedder AM. MRA of the thoracic vessels. *Semin Ultrasound CT MR* 2003; **24**:192–216.

13. Prince MR, Schoenberg SO, Ward JS et al. Hemodynamically significant atherosclerotic renal artery stenosis: MR angiographic features. *Radiology* 1997; **205**:128–36.

14. Ruehm SG, Hany TF, Pfammatter T et al. Pelvic and lower extremity arterial imaging: diagnostic performance of three-dimensional contrast-enhanced MR angiography. *AJR* 2000; **174**:1127–35.

15. Runge VM, Knopp MV. Off-label use and reimbursement of contrast media in MR. *JMRI* 1999; **10**:489–95.

16. Shellock FG, Kanal E. Safety of magnetic resonance imaging contrast agents. *J Magn Reson Imaging* 1999; **10**:477–84.

17. Runge VM. Safety of approved MR contrast media for intravenous injection. *J Magn Reson Imaging* 2000; **12**:205–13.

18. Mathur-de Vré R, Lemort M. Biophysical properties and clinical applications of magnetic resonance imaging contrast agents. *Br J Radiol* 1995; **68**:225–47.

19. Haustein J, Niendorf H, Krestin G et al. Renal tolerance of gadolinium-DTPA dimeglumine in patients with chronic renal failure. *Invest Radiol* 1992; **27**:153–6.

20. Bellin MF, Deray G, Assogba U et al. Gd-DOTA: evaluation of its renal tolerance in patients with chronic renal failure. *Magn Reson Imaging* 1992; **10**:115–18.

21. Bellin MF, Vasile M, Morel-Precetti S. Currently used non-specific extracellular MR contrast media. *Eur Radiol* 2003; **13**:2688–98.

22. Yoshikawa K, Davies A. Safety of ProHance in special population. *Eur Radiol* 1997; **7(Suppl 5)**: 246–50.

23. Tombach B, Bremer C, Reimer P et al. Using highly concentrated gadobutrol as an MR contrast agent in patients also requiring hemodialysis: safety and dialysability. *AJR* 2002; **178**:105–9.

24. Bartels LW, Bakker CJG. Endovascular interventional magnetic resonance imaging. *Phys Med Biol* 2003; **48**:R37–R64.

25. Godart F, Beregi JP, Nicol L et al. MR-guided balloon angioplasty of stenosed aorta: in vivo evaluation using near-standard instruments and a passive tracking technique. *J Magn Reson Imaging* 2000; **12**:639–44.

26. Manke C, Nitz WR, Djavidani B et al. MR imaging-guided stent placement in iliac arterial stenoses: a feasibility study. *Radiology* 2001; **219**:527–34.

27. Bilecen D, Schulte AC, Heidecker HG et al. Lower extremity: low-dose contrast agent intraarterial MR angiography in patients – initial results. *Radiology* 2005; **234**:250–5.

28. Wacker FK, Reither K, Ebert W et al. MR image-guided endovascular procedures with the ultrasmall superparamagnetic iron oxide SH U 555 C as an intravascular contrast agent: study in pigs. *Radiology* 2003; **226**:459–64.

29. Serfaty JM, Yang X, Foo TK et al. MRI-guided coronary catheterization and PTCA: a feasibility study on a dog model. *Magn Reson Med* 2003; **49**:258–63.

30. Kerns SR, Hawkins IF. Carbon dioxide digital subtraction angiography: expanding application and technical evolution. *AJR* 1995; **164**:735–41.

31. Solomon R, Werner C, Mann V et al. Effects of saline, mannitol and furosemide to prevent acute disease in renal function induced by radiocontrast agents. *N Engl J Med* 1994; **331**:1416–20.

32. Harkonen S, Kjellstrand C. Exacerbation of diabetic renal failure following intravenous pyelography. *Am J Med* 1977; **63**:939.

33. Parfrey PS, Griffiths SM, Barrett BJ et al. Contrast material induced renal failure in patients with diabete mellitus: renal insufficiency or both. *N Engl J Med* 1989; **320**:143–53.

34. Hawkins IF, Caridi JG. Carbon dioxide (CO_2) digital subtraction angiography: 26 year experience at the university of Florida. *Eur Radiol* 1998; **8**:391–402.

35. Hawkins IF. Carbon dioxide: digital subtraction angiography. *AJR* 1982; **139**:19–24.

36. Bettman MA, D'Agostino R, Jurawsky LI et al. Carbon dioxide as an angiographic contrast agent: a prospective randomized trial. *Invest Radiol* 1994; **29**:S45–S46.

37. Yang X, Manninen H, Soimakallio S. Carbon dioxide in vascular imaging and intervention. *Acta Radiol* 1995; **36**:330–7.

38. Seeger JM, Self M, Haward TRS et al. Carbon dioxide gas as an arterial contrast agent. *Ann Surg* 1993; **217**:688–98.

39. Oliva V, Common A, Bettmann MA et al. Prospective randomized crossover pilot study of the safety and efficacy of carbon dioxide versus iodinated contrast for peripheral angiography. *Acad Radiol* 1998; **5(Suppl 1)**:S58–S59.

40. Thomson KR, Tello R, Sullivan R et al. Carbon dioxide angiography. *Oceanian J Radiol* 1996; **1**:20–3.

41. Paúl L, Pínto I, Alfayate J et al. Assessment of CO_2 arteriography in arterial occlusive disease of the lower extremities. *JVIR* 2000; **11**:163–9.

42. Rolland Y, Duvauferrier R, Lucas A et al. Lower limb angiography: a prospective study comparing carbon dioxide with iodinated contrast material in 30 patients. *AJR* 1998; **171**:333–7.

43. Rundback JH, Shah PM, Wong J et al. Livedo reticularis, rhabdomyolysis, massive intestinal infarction and death after carbon dioxide arteriography. *J Vasc Surg* 1997; **26**:337–40.

44. Beese RC, Beese NR, Belli AM. Renal angiography using carbon dioxide. *Br J Radiol* 2000; **73**:3–6.

45. Schreier DZ, Weaver FA, Frankhouse J et al. A prospective study of carbon dioxide-DSA vs standard contrast arteriography in the evaluation of the renal arteries. *Arch Surg* 1996; **131**:503–7.

46. Kessel DO, Robertson I, Patel JV et al. Carbon-dioxide-guided vascular interventions: technique and pitfalls. *Cardiovasc Interven Radiol* 2002; **25**:476–83.

47. Weaver FA, Pentecost MJ, Yellin AE et al. Clinical applications of carbon dioxide/digital subtraction angiography. *J Vasc Surg* 1991; **13**:266–73.

48. Eschelmann DJ, Sullivan KL, Bonn J et al. Carbon dioxide as a contrast agent to guide vascular interventional procedures. *AJR* 1998; **171**:1265–70.

49. Burke CT, Weeks SM, Mauro MA et al. CO$_2$ splenoportography for evaluating the splenic and portal veins before and after liver transplantation. *J Vasc Interven Radiol* 2004; **15**:1161–5.

50. Caridi JG, Hawkins IF, Cho K. CO$_2$ splenoportography: preliminary results. *AJR* 2003; **180**:1375–8.

51. Rees CR, Niblett RL, Lee SP et al. Use of carbon dioxide as a contrast medium for transjugular intrahepatic portosystemic shunt procedures. *J Vasc Interven Radiol* 1994; **5**:383–6.

INDEX

N.B. *Italics* denote material appearing in figures or tables but not in the main body of text